Praise for *Subliminal Thera*

D0084473

The process of therapy presented by Dr. Yager is not to be confused with subliminal messages of old. It appears to result in a hypnotic state without a formal induction or use of typical hypnotic suggestions. Instead, the person is guided through a step-by-step process that is modifiable for use for many differing conditions. The process is "client-centered" with a strong reliance on the patient's own resources. Without the included case illustrations and results from evaluations, the technique might seem preposterous, particularly to those well-entrenched in a mental health practice based on better known principles and methods.

The book will challenge your beliefs about the basis of mental and physical behavior and dysfunctional conditions with findings and principles that are thought-provoking, if not convincing. This work of innovation and devotion will help you learn a technique, supported by evidence of rather remarkable benefit for several conditions. It would seem only a matter of time before treatment of many medical disorders is based on the principles and techniques proposed here, aiming more directly at the cause and with more use of the person's own resources.

James H. Stewart, MD, Mayo Clinic in Florida

Edwin Yager is a highly respected clinical hypnotherapist and this excellent book describes subliminal techniques which can be used with or without normal trance induction to help in discovering the roots of present-day presenting problems, where those suffering have been unable to uncover their cause. The book is written with great clarity and detail and will, I am certain, be of enormous benefit to practicing therapists whether or not they have already been contemplating the use of subliminal therapy in the treatment of those who consult them.

Ursula Markham, Founder and Principal of the Hypnothink Foundation

This book grabbed my attention in the very first paragraph of the Prologue by mentioning how two sessions of subliminal therapy resulted in a client's asthma ceasing, with no recurring symptoms after 39 months. The author's work developing Subliminal Therapy (ST) is innovative and brilliant, and it spans almost four decades.

Since much of health-care today helps patients and/or clients deal with the effects of physical or mental problems, it is very significant that the author resolves causes rather than just treating the symptoms. He states: "Resolve the *cause* and the problem goes away, not just temporarily, it goes away, period."

Actual case histories are presented to document the results. Examples include smoking cessation, anxiety, pain reduction, anger management, alcohol abuse, panic attacks, and more. Success rates were measured. The overall success rate for ST averages more than 80 percent, with a profound success rate of 94 percent for addictions. One category with a lower success, pain reduction, still reflects an impressive 75 percent success rate.

The author works on the concept that the mind contains a conscious, a subconscious, and a higher level of unconscious functioning that he calls "Centrum". This extra-consciousness is aware of various parts of the mind (also called ego states, or selves); and awareness of the subconscious parts is employed during the sessions. However, ST differs from both Ego State Therapy and Parts Therapy, because the facilitator communicates with Centrum rather than with the parts. Centrum then communicates directly with the parts at the facilitator's request, educating and/or persuading the client's parts, and indicating when the work is complete.

Flow charts appear in the appendices to ensure certain protocols are employed by anyone using ST. Additionally, in order to provide proper training in ST to health-care professionals, the author offers training and certification through the Subliminal Therapy Institute, Inc., in Southern California.

Whether or not one wishes to use Subliminal Therapy, I recommend that health-care professionals and hypnotherapists alike read this book.

C. Roy Hunter, PhD, FAPHP, author of several hypnosis texts, including *Hypnosis for Inner Conflict Resolution: Introducing Parts Therapy*

Dr. Yager's Subliminal Therapy presents a fresh challenge to conventional theories of disturbance. His understanding of the concept of a divided mind that incorporates a higher intelligence called Centrum is intriguing and will spark interest in anyone involved in the psychotherapeutic treatment of psychological, psychogenic and physical conditions. The refreshingly liberal use of case histories throughout gives the reader a true taste for, and confidence in, the clear and rational structured approach that is Subliminal Therapy.

Peter Mabbutt, FBSCH, FBAMH, CEO/Director of Studies, London College of Clinical Hypnosis

The dedication in Dr. Yager's *Subliminal Therapy* is telling: "to those clinicians ... who have the intellectual curiosity to seek improved ways to help people, the openness to consider that which is truly new and the willingness to test the effectiveness of the techniques they use." This is a book that ticks many boxes: being truly ground-breaking, yet highly practical; imaginative, yet rigorously researched; and accessible, yet intellectually satisfying.

Drawing on forty years experience of employing hypnotic procedures in psychotherapy, Yager clearly demonstrates how the methods and protocols of Subliminal Therapy – utilizing hypnotic techniques without requiring a formal trance induction – can be used to facilitate both psychological *and* physical healing.

Theoretical material is well-supported by extensive case material, which demonstrates Yager's pioneering work in the application of the psychology of mind–body healing.

In common with Griffin and Tyrrell's *Human Givens*, this is a book which expands its readers' understanding of the enormous potential of trance-work and reframing for achieving therapeutic ends in their broadest sense.

I highly recommend it.

John Perry, MA, MA, MSc, FHEA, Principal Teaching Fellow in Healthcare Communication, University of Southampton, UK

Subliminal Therapy

Subliminal Therapy

Using the Mind to Heal

Edwin K. Yager, Ph.D.

Crown House Publishing Limited
www.crownhouse.co.uk
www.crownhousepublishing.com

First published by

Crown House Publishing Ltd
Crown Buildings, Bancyfelin, Carmarthen, Wales, SA33 5ND, UK
www.crownhouse.co.uk

and

Crown House Publishing Company LLC
6 Trowbridge Drive, Suite 5, Bethel, CT 06801-2858, USA
www.crownhousepublishing.com

British Library Cataloguing-in-Publication Data
A catalogue entry for this book is available
from the British Library.

Print ISBN 978-184590-728-0
Mobi ISBN 978-184590-764-8
epub ISBN 978-184590-765-5
LCCN 2011928285

Printed and bound in the USA

This book is dedicated to those clinicians, both established and new to the field, who have the intellectual curiosity to seek improved ways to help people, the openness to consider that which is truly new and the willingness to test the effectiveness of the techniques they use.

Prologue

TJ, a 22-year-old female, presented with a twenty-plus year history of asthma that had not responded to traditional treatment. Following two one-hour treatment sessions by Subliminal Therapy, all symptoms of asthma had ceased. And after thirty-nine months, no symptoms have recurred.

This case illustrates the unique effectiveness of Subliminal Therapy, as do the following two cases:

LV presented with a forty-year history of unremitting pain. LV, now 64, was in an air crash during the Vietnam War in which he suffered damage to the bones and nerves of his upper body, shoulders and neck. He had been in severe pain since that experience and was living with a morphine drip. Following three hours of treatment by Subliminal Therapy, he reported 88 percent relief, with 90 percent relief reported two months post-treatment and maintained an additional forty-four months post-treatment. His morphine drip is now at one-fourth the dose at the beginning of treatment.

HJ, 34, presented with panic attacks, experienced on a daily basis for many years that had not responded either to pharmacology or to psychotherapy treatment. The attacks totally remitted after four hours of treatment by Subliminal Therapy and have not recurred twenty-four months post-treatment.

These cases are not unique in the application of Subliminal Therapy. They are not even unusual and are in fact quite common. By using Subliminal Therapy, clinicians are capable of providing lasting cure of psychogenic disorders and of providing marked relief from pain and emotional distress in consequence of physical trauma, as well as physical diseases such as cancer.

Subliminal Therapy predates the practice of reframing as described by Bandler and Grinder (1983) and offers a more extensive protocol for actually resolving the underlying causes of psychogenic disorders. The intellectual capacities of the patient are utilized in the process, tapping into commonly unrecognized abilities, abilities that might be described as extra-conscious, doing so using a rational, logical protocol.

Subliminal Therapy is not just an idealized dream. The technique was developed almost forty years ago and has been researched on a continual basis. Data has been accumulated during recent years to substantiate its effectiveness, data that is presented herein. This book, coupled with exposure to video recordings of the application of Subliminal Therapy, will prepare you, the established clinician, to help your patients in ways just as dramatic as the cases above, and will introduce these concepts to those new to the helping professions.

Preface

During forty years of studying and employing hypnotic techniques, I have come to several clearly defined conclusions. The clearest of these is that we have mental capacities far beyond those we currently comprehend. In particular, we have capacities to heal both mentally and physically, and to do so with efficiency and thoroughness that we have only begun to understand. I believe Subliminal Therapy is a forerunner of psychotherapeutic techniques to accomplish such healing.

We do, of course, already know *some* remarkable things. We know of our capacity to achieve anesthesia without chemical aid. We know of our mental ability to either accelerate or to impede the healing of wounds. We strongly suspect the role of mental influence in the causes of some illnesses that have classically been considered in the realm of physical origin. I have personally witnessed healing of some aspects of traumatic brain injury unexplained by conventional standards. I have witnessed progress in improving some symptoms of autism and of the cure of many cases of asthma, all by the intervention of mental capacities.

Another clearly defined conclusion I have reached is that a large percentage of *physical* illnesses that plague humankind are, in fact, psychogenic. This conclusion is not original; we have long recognized the influence of emotional and mental states on many disorders. Gastro-intestinal, dermatological and respiratory illnesses are illustrations; to extrapolate our thoughts into the domain of 'cause' is not unreasonable. The action of smooth muscle, controlled by unconscious processes, can affect all physical processes by occluding airways and arteries and by altering glandular secretions. If such action were to disturb physical processes, creating the symptoms of an illness, although prompted by an emotional disturbance, it would be diagnosed as organic illness.

In this book I offer a systematic protocol, *Subliminal Therapy*, which has proven successful as an effective treatment by purely mental intervention, of a surprisingly wide variety of presenting problems, both mental and physical. The assumptions upon which this protocol is based range from being conventionally logical to stretching the credibility of many clinicians. I recall the reaction of one psychologist when he was first exposed to the Subliminal Therapy protocol as he uttered, "What unmitigated nonsense!" As the reader of this book, you might conceivably, at least initially, have a similar reaction. It is my hope that you will test the validity of Subliminal Therapy for yourself. You will find it sound.

I recognize that the theory of human mental functioning I present here is at odds with the conventional psychiatric model, in which mental illness is believed to be the *consequence* of chemical imbalance in the brain. Instead, I believe the chemical imbalance is the consequence of the mental illness. There is no question that chemical imbalance exists in mental disorders; it is the cause–effect relationship between them that I see as reversed. For example, in conventional psychiatry, depression is considered to be the consequence of chemical imbalance, and the DSM diagnostic criteria is based upon that assumption. In opposition, I consider depression to be the consequence of conditioning from life experiences, and the preferred treatment is therefore by mental intervention, not by medication. The accuracy of my position on this matter is demonstrated in the data on the success rates of Subliminal Therapy (see Chapter VI).

Contents

Introduction

This is a 'how to' book. In reading these pages, I will introduce you to Subliminal Therapy (ST) and teach you the procedures involved in applying the technique. I will make you aware of the potential ST has to literally cure or effectively ease the trauma of many disorders, some physical as well as many psychological.

As presented in this book, I do not view ST to be the final form or the final word about the technique. During the course of development, ST has evolved in form and organization, and I anticipate it will continue to evolve as insights beyond my own are contributed. For example, the concept of Centrum, as introduced in Chapter I, is the least understood of the premises of ST, and I am satisfied that Centrum has capabilities not yet explored. I urge readers to explore them on their own. It is already evident that Centrum has unexplained capabilities in the domain of pain control, tumor remission, dissociative disorders and immunization – and these are just the beginning.

The concept of ST evolved from my 'engineering' way of thinking. Even before I left my career in electronic engineering, I became interested in hypnotic phenomena and the unconscious capacities that a patient in trance could access. The essential concepts of ST are rooted in hypnotic phenomena, and I therefore consider it be a hypnotic technique. Both conscious thought and subconscious thought have levels of complexity and awareness and the concept of the existence of a higher level of unconscious functioning evolved as I struggled to explain the way humans function. We are conditioned creatures, and if that conditioning results in the creation of 'learned' elements of our mental functioning, and these elements are represented in the unconscious domain as separate influences, how are we able to function in organized ways, rather than being dysfunctional, with our attention and direction randomly dictated by the influences of the moment? My answer was that there has to be a higher level of cognitive or psychological functioning, and with the many hundreds of patients with whom I have used ST, that higher level of functioning has been apparent in almost every one of them. In 1974 I named that level of the subconscious domain 'Centrum'.

As a clinician, I greatly prefer to identify and resolve the cause of a problem, rather than wrestle with its symptoms. When cause is resolved, symptoms cease to exist. Not only can treatment result in curing the problem, meaning permanent resolution, it is also the most time-efficient approach available. The success rates quoted in Chapter IV summarize the self-evaluations of patients I have treated in the recent past, as documented by patient-completed inventories.

I conceive humanity as being conditioned by life-experiences, and the effects of conditioning can endure for a lifetime. It is through conditioning that we learn values, skills, behaviors and limitations. Sometimes we also learn dysfunctional values, skills, behaviors and limitations.

Conditioned responses may become subconscious responses, and there is seldom conscious awareness of the etiology of a resultant problem. Phobic persons do not know why they are phobic, and the person with migraine headaches does not know why they occur. A great many presenting problems are the consequence of conditioning and a common denominator is their manifestation through the misguided action of smooth muscle. Misguided, that is, by the controlling, subconscious mental process that is, in turn, the consequence of experience.

The action of smooth muscle maintains life itself by modulating glandular function, digestion, respiration and the pattern of blood flow in the body, all controlled via the autonomic nervous system. If misguided, such action may manifest as an asthma attack, a migraine headache, a gastro-intestinal or dermatological problem. And, since the action of smooth muscle can be controlled by mental processes, and subconscious process is determined by conditioning, is it not apparent that some physical illnesses can be psychogenic, as psychosomatic medicine has so long maintained?

Chapter I

Background and Concepts

In this chapter I present the concept of Subliminal Therapy from conception through its evolution. After an overview of the technique, I present its clinical acceptance, structure, advantages, limitations and appropriate areas of application.

Origin of the Concept of Subliminal Therapy

I first conceived the technique I named Subliminal Therapy (ST) in 1974. As with all developments in our field, the concept evolved from knowledge of the work of others who I will duly acknowledge. At that time I had transitioned from a career in engineering into the world of psychotherapy and was applying my engineering way of thinking to explain human behavior as I had learned about it in my studies and through personal observations. I noticed that consistent, conscious self-control of behavior, a concept I had accepted as reality, was an illusion. Undesired thoughts, habits and behaviors of many kinds are commonly and repeatedly experienced against our will. In spite of our cultural admonition to be in conscious control, I recognized that subconscious functioning is the locus of control.

Moreover, I came to recognize that the subconscious domain is not a unified whole as conventionally regarded; instead it is sub-divided, with distinctively different parts representing learned beliefs, skills, limitations, personality traits, values and behaviors that are sometimes in conflict with each other. This fact, I came to understand, was the root of many problems that my patients presented. I also understood that these parts were created in the course of life experiences, i.e., they were conditioned responses. This concept of a divided subconscious is not

1

new. I found similarities with Ego State Therapy by Watkins (1979), Freud (1938) and within the principles taught by Jung (1916, 1933).

It seems that when an experience occurs and a lesson is learned, a new part of the mind is created. 'Something' is present in the subconscious domain now, something that was not there before the experience occurred. This something may manifest consciously in the form of emotion or compulsive behavior; however, conscious awareness of the influences prompting the emotion or behavior is rarely present. This subconscious part represents the learning that occurred in the course of the experience and may thereafter continue to play an active role in the person's life, maintaining the theme of the original lesson. For example: If a child learns he is stupid – as might happen if he is called stupid by a person seen as an authority – the part of his mind that was created in that situation may continue to influence his life by compromising his self-image. He may also continue to behave stupidly based on the subconscious belief that he *is* stupid. On the other hand, if the lesson is positive, such as, "You are smart," the part created continues to influence his life in positive ways. The accumulation of a multitude of such parts, each derived from life experiences, seems to constitute a major portion of the subconscious domain, with the balance representing genetic and perhaps spiritual factors. Also, reinforcing experiences or conflicting experiences create reinforcing or conflicting parts. This way of thinking about the mind is fundamental to the concept of ST. In this model of the mind, therapy consists of identifying the problematic parts and then reconditioning them to support the current needs and values of the individual and society.

In the model of the mind upon which Subliminal Therapy is based, three levels of mental functioning are apparent: *Consciousness*, the *Subconscious* domain and a level of *Extra-Conscious* capability. The similar construct of Freudian psychoanalysis comes to mind, corresponding to the Id, Ego and Super-Ego. However, in Subliminal Therapy the work of therapy is accomplished in the extra-conscious domain, while in psychoanalysis the work is accomplished consciously.

Our *conscious* abilities are at once awesome and limited. On the awesome side, there is love, creativity and intelligence. On the limited side, we commonly hold an exaggerated expectation of our ability to control ourselves. We envision abilities to make desired changes that are quite beyond our capacity to execute. Examples include abilities to self-cure phobias, compulsions and irrational convictions, as well as limitations typically recognized as irrational, yet that continue in spite of the exertion of conscious will.

The *subconscious* domain seems to be the repository of influences from life experiences and totally lacking in the ability to be proactive. This domain is analogous to the random access memory of a computer: it is subject to change and motivated to action in response to outside stimulus, and it provides data to associated functions such as speech, yet it is not capable of self-initiated action. It is intelligent only in the sense that it is capable of learning and relearning. Importantly, it is the domain that is (conditionally) subject to the influence of direct hypnotic suggestions.

The *extra-conscious* mind, on the other hand, seems to have self-awareness. That domain has the ability to 'think' in the same way that we think consciously, i.e., to reason, to relate cause and effect, and to extrapolate. The extra-conscious domain usually possesses a sense of the value of the self and is willing to cooperate in improving the status of the self. I cannot explain how a person could function normally without a unifying – and perhaps guiding – influence in the subconscious domain. Such an influence must provide direction and purpose, as well as facilitate communication among these sub-divided elements I refer to as 'parts'. This seems to be the role of the extra-conscious domain, to which I initially assigned the name 'Control'. However, I shortly realized a different name was needed, since 'Control' was factually a misnomer (arbitrary control does not seem to exist there), and I have since used the name 'Centrum'.

I cannot objectively validate Centrum as an entity, as opposed to a hypothetical construct, to the satisfaction of a determined skeptic. I can, however, validate Centrum to the subjective

3

satisfaction of my patients and myself. And, after interacting with the Centrums of several thousand patients, I have reached subjective conviction of its validity. It is clear to me that there is a higher level of intelligence in all of us, an entity that is positively disposed toward our wellbeing. On more than one occasion patients have affirmed Centrum as their "Soul". I am satisfied that it does not really matter what name is applied. Validation of Centrum occurs in the process in which Centrum is engaged to accomplish the desired change. Patients may initially express reservations; however, as soon as the process has begun, and Centrum has demonstrated its existence, patients cease to raise questions.

The Clinical Acceptance of Subliminal Therapy

Early in its development, I was concerned about the model of Subliminal Therapy being too unconventional or too unusual to be accepted as legitimate by mainstream psychotherapists. Such acceptance was never a problem with my patients; they were participating with enthusiasm. Professionals, on the other hand, did not have the full picture; they were typically exposed to only the basic theory of ST without the benefit of personal experience or validation by clinical trials.

My concerns were based in reality; even today a few clinicians continue to regard Subliminal Therapy as bizarre and too far outside the mainstream. On the other hand, I have trained psychologists, masters-level therapists, medical students and physicians in its use, doing so without the unconventionality barrier being a problem. As its reputation expands and research data has accumulated, ST has experienced broader acceptance, and those clinicians familiar with its use are vocal in promoting its concepts. Insofar as patients are concerned, while a few may have reservations initially, and some may be too polite to express those reservations, few of them maintain those reservations when the stage has been set and therapy has begun.

I believe we will see broader clinical acceptance only as research data affirms the effectiveness of ST, and such research has not yet occurred to the degree necessary. Yet data are gradually accumulating, and this unconventional approach to personal change is being affirmed as the outstanding, effective and efficient technique I know it to be.

Overview of the Process

In this segment of the book, I divide the process of Subliminal Therapy into five phases, describing each phase and providing flow charts in Appendix A to guide clinicians in learning its application.

Phase I

Phase I consists of building rapport with the patient, educating the patient about the technique and clarifying the goal(s) of therapy. This phase typically requires thirty minutes to an hour, depending upon the skill of the therapist, as well as the patient's openness to new concepts. The time may be shortened if the patient has had previous exposure to ST, either via the Internet (e.g., via my website, www.docyager.com) or by having read *Subliminal Therapy: Utilizing Subconscious Abilities in Therapy* (Yager, 1999), a booklet I created for the purpose of introducing the concepts to patients.

Phase II

This phase consists of establishing communication with the patient's Centrum, determining Centrum's willingness to support the conscious goal and clarifying Centrum's ability to do the necessary work. This phase typically consumes less than ten minutes. However, in a small percentage of cases Centrum must be educated about essential capabilities, in which case an hour or more may be required.

Phase III

Phase III is beginning the application of Subliminal Therapy to the presenting problem. Here the flowcharts may be of great aid to the clinician who is learning the technique (see Chapter III and Appendix A). Centrum is engaged and guided to take the necessary steps. The knowledge and clinical training of the therapist is focused on executing a rational decision tree that is at once challenging and satisfying, both to the clinician and to the patient. The concepts presented above are subjectively experienced by the patient, with real validation of the technique occurring as desired change takes place in real world experiences.

Phase IV

This is a process of determining if the work is as complete as possible at this time. Is there more to be done? Is there some remaining issue that has not yet been recognized, an issue that might cause the problem to continue? If there is any indication that an additional issue exists, it must be addressed. If no further issues appear to exist, such indication is still not absolute; the ultimate test of completeness lies in the real world as the patient experiences everyday life. Nevertheless, these steps are valuable in providing immediate, if not a final, indication of remaining issues that must be resolved.

Note: Completing Phases III and IV may require less than an hour, or may require multiple hours, typically averaging from two to four hours, including the initial hour of history-taking and evaluation.

Phase V

Follow-up. In some cases, in spite of all available indications that the work of therapy has been completed, the problem continues after the patient leaves the session. It may continue at a less severe level, or even at a greater level of severity, or rarely in modified form. Nevertheless, in such cases further work is required, and the concern is that the patient might conclude "It isn't working" and withdraw from treatment. It is important for the patient to recognize that recurrence of the problem simply indicates the work is not complete, as opposed to the work not having been successful. Should the problem continue, explain that some other part remains, some part not previously recognized, that is actively causing the problem to continue and that additional therapy can resolve the problem entirely. You should assure them that immediate continuation of the problem does not indicate failure, either by them or the technique. A legitimate conclusion of failure of ST applies when no subconscious cause can be found and the problem continues.

Comparison of Subliminal Therapy to Other Therapeutic Techniques

Clinicians have many therapeutic techniques available to choose from. All, including ST, incorporate hypnotic phenomena either overtly or covertly, with or without the intention or awareness of the clinician. I have presented a few techniques in the following paragraphs and have contrasted them with ST as a means of explaining ST more fully. Since ST is essentially a psychodynamic technique, I have only presented psychodynamic techniques for comparison.

Psychoanalysis

In psychoanalysis, the patient is encouraged to consciously explore psychogenic variables by means of free association and other techniques with the objective of achieving insight into the factors causing the presenting problem. This insight is then interpreted by the analyst to arrive at new understanding, which is then integrated by the patient.

Subliminal Therapy

In marked contrast, conscious involvement in the process of therapy is minimized; the work is accomplished by the patient's extra-conscious abilities (Centrum). As opposed to insight (which is a necessary but insufficient component), in ST the analysis and interpretation of uncovered material is accomplished by the *patient* without involvement of outside opinion; the therapist acts as a guide of the process with only occasional involvement in the content of the work.

Hypnotic Age Regression

In this technique, the therapist utilizes the enhanced ability to recall information that is afforded by the trance state to identify life experiences that have resulted in dysfunctional current behaviors. Then the therapist typically evaluates and reframes the retrieved information with the goal of eliminating the dysfunction. The patient is consciously aware of, and involved in the steps in the process and may accomplish evaluation and reframing independently of the therapist.

Subliminal Therapy

Two primary differences are apparent: In Hypnotic Age Regression there is no recognition of extra-conscious abilities and no recognition of the sub-divided nature of the subconscious domain. By utilizing ST, the therapist avoids the interfering bias of the patient's conscious opinions and recognizes greater time efficiency.

The Analytical Use of Ideo-Motor Responses

As taught by LeCron (1965), Cheek (1994) and Ewin (2006), the use of ideo-motor responses, commonly in the form of finger signals, to perceive communications from the subconscious domain, has proven effective in a great many cases by many different clinicians. LeCron defined the *Seven Keys*, questions that were of a specific nature, questions that expedited identification of the underlying causes of current problems. The subconscious domain is typically regarded as being unified, and questions are posed in that context. The technique also assumes capabilities of the subconscious domain that are beyond just a memory bank.

Subliminal Therapy

The ideo-motor approach to treatment lacks the time efficiency of ST because the answers from Centrum are limited to the coded meaning assigned to the fingers, as opposed to the use of a chalkboard or inner voice which avoids that limitation. To be sure, the use of the chalkboard could be incorporated instead of the finger signals to perceive communications; however, the greater difference lies in the concept of engaging extra-conscious abilities to achieve the desired change, as elaborated in the following chapters.

Subconscious Guided Therapy

Anbar (2008) described an efficient extension of automatic writing while the patient is in trance, utilizing a computer with two keyboards, one for the patient's subconscious and one for the therapist. On one keyboard the therapist types questions to be answered by the subconscious mind of the patient, which, in turn, is typing on the other keyboard using the fingers of the patient. When using this technique, the patient may be consciously aware of the information on the computer screen but is often unaware of typing his/her contribution.

Subliminal Therapy

This new and promising technique (SGT) utilizes subconscious abilities for therapeutic purposes, as does ST, but fails to recognize the sub-divided nature of subconscious functioning and the existence of extra-conscious abilities. In Subconscious Guided Therapy, the therapist does not recognize that subconscious influence may be influential in causing problems, assuming instead that the received communications are fully informed and authoritative. ST, on the other hand, makes no such assumptions; the team of therapist and patient investigate and uncover possible influences that are then resolved in a more comprehensive and structured way (see Chapter III).

Additionally, ST utilizes extra-conscious abilities that may not have been recognized by the patient, those that Centrum represents. These abilities are resident in everyone, and the rational, logical, pragmatic way in which ST utilizes them sets it apart from other therapeutic techniques.

Ego State Therapy

As conceived by Watkins (1993), this technique recognizes the dissociative qualities and characteristics of the subconscious domain and the existence of discrete 'ego states'. The therapist interacts with these ego states individually to resolve the patient's issues. The therapist also employs traditional psychotherapy techniques of treatment (hypnotic and otherwise) in interacting with each ego state, as with individual patients using conventional techniques.

Subliminal Therapy

ST also recognizes the sub-divided nature of the subconscious domain, addresses the individual components and resolves their influences. However, in ST this task is accomplished by Centrum, sometimes without conscious awareness of the work in progress, making possible a far more efficient and thorough resolution of the presenting problem because conscious rational bias is bypassed.

The Inner Advisor

John Bresler (1990) conceived this intervention. It is an insight-oriented, hypnotherapeutic technique used to uncover information related to presenting symptoms and assumes the existence of inner wisdom (communicated from an inner advisor). Carl Jung's (1916) theory of personality supports this inner wisdom concept and this approach is receiving increasing attention in industry literature. The inner advisor is usually represented by an imagined animal; however, it may be in human form.

Subliminal Therapy

This technique differs from ST in multiple ways, including lack of recognition of a sub-divided subconscious, as well as lack of recognition of abilities such as those exhibited by Centrum. The goal of uncovering causal information is the primary common factor. Additionally, ST makes no assumption that Centrum is *wise*, as in the case of the Inner Advisor. Rather, Centrum is assumed to be *intelligent* and to have abilities not available consciously.

Parts Therapy

Jung (1916) proposed the concept of the subconscious domain being made up of multiple 'parts'. As formalized by Roy Hunter (2005), Parts Therapy reconciles conflicting parts of the subconscious mind by engineering negotiation between the parts, through the therapist, with the objective of resolving the problem.

Subliminal Therapy

Although the Parts Therapy model recognizes the sub-divided nature of the subconscious domain, the application differs from ST in several ways. Parts Therapy directly and fully involves the clinician in the *content* of the work as it progresses and does not recognize or utilize the higher level of functioning represented by Centrum. Instead, the 'wisdom' obtained from the subconscious is used to guide conscious action. In ST, Centrum is not necessarily accredited with wisdom. Instead, Centrum may have knowledge not available to consciousness, thereby appearing wise; however, Centrum has not accessed the pool of universal knowledge proposed by Jung. Actually, the range of Centrum's knowledge has not been defined. There are occasional indications during therapy sessions that Centrum has some sort of unexpected awareness of instinctual and functional processes; however, no research into this domain has been accomplished.

Psychosynthesis

Assagioli (1965) conceived Psychosynthesis as an essential way of thinking about psychotherapy, a way that can embrace many specific techniques and modes. The aim of Psychosynthesis is generalized, but primarily seeks to develop the whole personality. This way of thinking involves cognitive process with full acknowledgment and development of the concept of subconscious functioning.

Subliminal Therapy

Beyond the lack of recognition of the higher level of functioning represented by Centrum, the most basic difference lies in the goals of treatment. ST focuses on specific problems, while the goal of Psychosynthesis is generalized. Also, ST is discretely organized and applied in a logical series of steps, while Psychosynthesis is broadly applied in a general way.

Voice Dialogue

Conceived by Hal and Sidra Stone in the late 1960s, and reaching its peak of popularity years later (Stone & Winkelman, 1989), as well as being allied to Ego State Therapy and Parts Therapy, this approach recognizes the existence of a multitude of 'selves' that collectively constitute our non-physical presentation, and understanding these selves as separate personalities.

Subliminal Therapy

In ST, the 'parts' of the subconscious mind are not understood as developed personalities. Rather, the individual parts are consistently limited in their awareness of the current life situation, instead functioning according to the influences present at the time of their conception. Also, Voice Dialogue does not acknowledge the existence or utilization of the higher level of intellectual functioning represented by Centrum.

PSYCH-K

In his book, *The Missing Peace In Your Life!*, Williams (2008) discusses an organization of the brain that more closely parallels ST than other therapies. He defines mental functioning as being *conscious*, *subconscious* and *superconscious* and describes the superconscious in ways similar to the way Centrum is described in ST. In PSYCH-K, the communication device of 'muscle testing' is employed to receive communications from the superconscious.

Subliminal Therapy

PSYCH-K does not envision the subconscious domain as being subdivided, as in ST. Nor does it recognize the capacities of extra-consciousness in identifying and resolving the causes of problems. In PSYCH-K, communication from subconsciousness to the therapist is limited to muscle testing, whereas in ST communication is verbal and flexible, possibly including any or all of the senses.

The strength of Subliminal Therapy lies in its rational structure and clarity in format and execution. It is a technique that makes it possible to actually resolve/eliminate/cure a problem, not just treat its symptoms. Moreover, ST works best when the clinician avoids assumptions regarding the etiology of the presenting problem, relying instead on the patient's extra-conscious ability to identify and to resolve the cause of problems, doing so with minimum involvement in the content of the information processed. Furthermore, the most conspicuous difference between Subliminal Therapy and the other techniques reviewed is the involvement of Centrum in the process of treatment.

Appropriate Treatment Applications

Subliminal Therapy is the treatment of choice for a wide variety of disorders that are psychogenic, and it is a valuable aid in the adjunctive treatment of many non-psychogenic disorders, especially in cases where emotion is an exacerbating influence. Moreover, in concert with psychosomatic research, I have come to believe a significant number of disorders that have classically been considered solely organic in etiology may in fact be psychogenic. Examples include Irritable Bowel Syndrome, Crohn's disease and asthma, disorders in which the mechanism of the problems is the action of smooth muscle, controlled in turn by subconscious processes, which in turn is influenced by emotion.

Practitioners commonly acknowledge that emotions produce physical reactions in the body; such reactions include changes in heart rate, blood pressure, blood chemistry, respiration, digestion and glandular function, as well as smooth and skeletal muscle tension. If the physiological reactions to a negative emotion such as fear were to continue in a protracted state over time, a clinician might diagnose the condition as an illness or disease without recognition of its true etiology.

Psychological Disorders

In ST, depression, anxiety, anger, grief and guilt are understood as symptoms of deeper problems, a concept at odds with the APA Diagnostic and Statistical Manual (DSM). Using ST, I have successfully treated all of the disorders listed in the DSM under the heading *Anxiety*, in addition to depression, addictions, dissociation, obsessions, compulsions and severe grief.

Note: In this book, I define "successfully treated" as meaning either total remission of symptoms, which is usually the case, or reduction in severity of the symptoms by at least 80 percent, both as reported by the patient. Symptom status is currently being reported by the patient by means of a brief, written inventory administered at the initial interview, immediately following treatment, and subsequently by follow-up inventories.

Physical Disorders of Psychogenic Origin

By using ST, I have successfully treated asthma, irritable bowel syndrome, vaginismus, erectile dysfunction, ulcers, psoriasis, migraine and tension headaches, many chronic and acute pain situations (notably low back pain), emesis associated with early pregnancy and some allergic reactions (e.g., to animals, other persons and situations).

All of these disorders are either psychogenic or exacerbated by psychological factors, and therefore all can be treated by psychological approaches. As a matter of safety of the patient, as well as legal protection for the therapist, the care of a physician is usually indicated; however, resolution of the psychogenic elements responsible for the presenting symptoms will consistently be required for full recovery. Those elements are products of conditioning, and resolution must involve reconditioning. Since reconditioning is the hallmark of intervention by ST, the use of ST is advocated.

Physical Disorders of Non-Psychogenic Origin

By using ST, I have successfully guided patients to relieve chronic and acute pain resulting from physical trauma, protracted pain without diagnosed physical cause, psychological components of chemical addictions and dyspepsia.

Regardless of their etiology, physical disorders can result in emotional reactions. If these emotional reactions have the consequence of inner tension, that tension may inhibit recovery in one or more ways. Possible examples include smooth muscle occlusion of arteries that restrict the flow of healing blood, an imbalance of blood chemistry inhibiting functioning of the immune system and the exacerbation of pain. Thus, psychological intervention can accelerate healing, ease discomfort and reduce the incidence of related disorders that are consequences of life experiences. ST has demonstrated extraordinary effectiveness in doing so.

Chapter II

Theory and Assumptions

In this chapter, I present the conceptual framework of Subliminal Therapy and the essential assumptions made in its derivation.

Subliminal Therapy is a technique in which subconscious cognitive abilities are accessed and utilized, i.e., abilities that are commonly not recognized consciously. By using this technique, the clinician can identify causal aspects of problems. Once identified, these problems can be resolved by considering their causes in the light of present, more mature and informed knowledge, as opposed to the limited knowledge and understanding in effect at the time when the causal influence began. The therapist utilizes the patient's present, mature understanding to alter or eliminate the influence of the original experience, by reconditioning by relearning, reframing or simply by reaching a different understanding about the cause.

The Underlying Principles of Subliminal Therapy

The following principles comprise the underpinnings of ST and are expanded upon in the following sections. These principles are rooted in the assumption that our mental processes occur in three domains: conscious, subconscious and extra-conscious.

- Our lives are largely determined by conditioning from experiences in life, whether from Pavlovian or operant conditioning. Values, beliefs and behaviors are all learned and can be relearned in a different way with different consequences provided certain conditions are met. Change will not happen unless these conditions are met:
  - We must be aware that it is possible to change conditioning.

- We must know how to accomplish the change.
- We must be motivated to do so.

- We have conscious awareness of only a very small part of our total mental functioning. Most of our mental capacity, as well as our mental functioning, takes place without conscious awareness.

- We possess a higher order of intelligence than we possess in the conscious domain, even though we are seldom taught how to recognize or to utilize it.

- Our subconscious domain is not a unified whole. Rather, it is fragmented, consisting of a great many parts – parts that represent the influences from past experiences. For example, when we learn a new skill, something is there now (in our mind) that was not there before. That something is referred to in ST as a 'part'. In similar form, if someone learns to fear spiders, that fear is represented by another newly formed part of the mind. Thus, a part may represent a skill, value, limitation or any other influence that was learned.

- These parts of the subconscious domain are the products of life experiences and may continue to exert the influence of those past experiences, even though to do so may be maladaptive and detrimental to the welfare of the person.

- We can influence (as opposed to command) these subconscious parts in desired ways by taking the following steps:
  - Recognize their existence.
  - Establish communication with them.
  - Educate them about current reality, needs and values, thereby persuading them to exert their influence in currently appropriate ways.

- Our higher-level mental capability, which for convenience I call Centrum, is in a position to communicate with, and to educate and influence, other subconscious parts. In utilizing these innate capacities, this higher-level ability is enlisted to assist in accomplishing consciously desired change.

The Assumptions of Subliminal Therapy

The superstructure of ST rests on four assumptions:

1. Intelligent, subconscious capability exists.

2. The subconscious domain can communicate with the conscious mind in identifiable ways.

3. The subconscious domain consists largely of subsystems, (parts) which may function autonomously.

4. There is an entity that may best be described as a 'higher intelligence' – an entity that is not well defined, yet is easily authenticated subjectively. This entity, which I have named Centrum, is described in Chapter I.

The First Assumption

Subconscious intelligence has been recognized by Cheek (1994), Erickson (1989a), Ewin (2006) and Watkins (1993) among many others:

> It is very important for a person to know their subconscious is smarter than they are. There is greater wealth of stored material in the subconscious. We know the subconscious can do things, and it is important to assure your patient that it can. They have to be willing to let their subconscious do things and not depend so much on their conscious mind. This is a great aid to their functioning. (Erickson & Rossi, 1976, p. 346)

In Subliminal Therapy, the therapist persuades patients to allow their subconscious minds to work in a logical, organized, sequential process, either through the guidance of the therapist or, under limited conditions, self-guided by the patient.

The Second Assumption

Centrum can communicate with the conscious mind, doing so in identifiable ways. In my classes I illustrate this communication by asking, "How do you spell cat?" I will point out that, although the students know how to spell 'cat', that was not on their minds before I asked the question. And, that since it was not on their minds, the answer had to have been communicated to consciousness from the subconscious domain. The letters were communicated to consciousness by one of the senses; perhaps they saw the letters, or perhaps they heard the letters. I will then ask for a show of hands as to which sense was engaged. I usually see slightly more "I saw them" hands than "I heard them" hands. Also, the phenomena of memory itself can be considered an illustration of subconscious-to-conscious communication in that information is perceived via visual, auditory or other senses.

The Third Assumption

The subconscious mind consists of multiple parts. The literature is rich with examples of recognition of the existence of such parts. Hilgard (1978a) states, "Personality is much less unified than we would like to believe and volition is subject to dissociation just as are perceptual processes." James's (1890) assertion that "Consciousness is split into parts that ignore each other," and Janet's (1907) interpretation that "Systems of ideas are split off from the major personality, subconscious but capable of becoming represented in consciousness through hypnosis," support this concept. Green and Green (1977) describe, "the autonomous entities working for themselves as subconscious parts of our psyche." Subliminal Therapy enlists these 'autonomous entities' for therapeutic purposes. Although I pointed out their differences in Chapter I, in respect to the concept of parts, ST is similar to Assagioli's Psychosynthesis (1965), which is described as a process of integration of the parts of the psyche, and to Watkins and Watkins's (1979) Ego State Therapy, in which various 'states' are 'cathected'.

18

The parts that constitute much, if not all, of the subconscious domain, seem limited in knowledge about the person and the world about them. They know only the information that pertained to the experience from which they were created. They lack 'personality' as a result of a complexity of factors. On the other hand, they are able to communicate directly with consciousness, as suggested by Watkins's Ego State Therapy.

The subconscious domain is made up of parts representing different ages and maturity levels, depending upon the stage of life in which they were conceived. Yet, all are intelligent, meaning that they are capable of learning, and all are disposed positively toward the welfare of the individual. However, they influence life in accordance with what *they* perceive to be advisable, which may be regarded by the patient as dysfunctional. In illustration, a part that is causing a conversion reaction is doing so in the best interests of the individual *as it perceives that best interest to be,* despite the opposing, conscious opinions of the patient.

The Fourth Assumption

The fourth assumption is that Centrum exists, an assumption not supported by reference to the literature with the exception of the work of Williams (2008). I originally assumed the existence of a higher level of subconscious functioning as an explanation for various phenomena I observed clinically, phenomena which defied other explanation. As the therapist engages the services of Centrum in the process of ST, communication takes place with the patient usually being consciously aware of the process, and the consistent beneficial outcome convincingly validates Centrum's existence.

As I conceive the organization of our minds, Centrum is simply a name for that higher order of intelligence. And yet, communicating with Centrum quickly impresses the clinician that Centrum has personality, a personality that usually, but not always, conforms with the personality of the patient. On occasion, Centrum has presented as being wholly separate from the patient, autonomously and indifferently directing events, but this situation is not common.

While usually consistent in presentation, Centrum may be of unexpected gender, or of no apparent gender, and may demonstrate changes in strengths and values as therapy proceeds.

Centrum can communicate with the patient at a conscious level of awareness and, through the patient, can communicate with the therapist. This inner-patient communication from Centrum to conscious awareness may be accomplished by means of ideo-motor signals, as classically described by Cheek (1994) in which coded meaning is assigned to the fingers. Other ideo-sensory means, such as an imagined chalkboard on which Centrum is requested to write, can be used, and by attending to an inner voice. Subjectively perceived physical sensations, as taught by Bandler and Grinder (1979), can also be coded as to meaning. Ewin (2006) has documented the viability of ideo-motor signals and Cheek and LeCron (1968) have described the use of finger signals and Chevreul's pendulum for that purpose. However, the most efficient way for Centrum to communicate with the therapist is by means of a chalkboard upon which Centrum can write, a chalkboard that is imagined by the patient. Especially for children, an imagined computer screen can be used in lieu of a chalkboard.

Since some may question the assumption of the existence of Centrum, I encourage the reader to personally test the assumption. For the moment, assume the possibility of the actuality of Centrum's existence, meaning that your Centrum does in fact exist and is capable of communicating with you at a conscious level. Pose a question to your Centrum by expressing it aloud, or by simply thinking it. Include a means whereby Centrum can respond, such as by writing on a chalkboard or indicating a physical sensation. For example, you might phrase your request as, *"Centrum, as a way of demonstrating your presence, please respond by a distinct inner voice, or by creating a distinct sensation some place in my body that can be repeated as needed to satisfy my critical judgment."*

In Summary

In Subliminal Therapy, the capacity for subconscious reasoning makes it possible to bypass much of the resistance typically evident in therapy. Moreover, should the therapist so choose, this capacity can free the therapist to conduct the course of therapy without necessarily being involved in the content being addressed by the patient. In a test of limits, I have successfully conducted therapy without even knowing the nature of the presenting problem (see Chapter VI). Even more startling, the patient may not be consciously aware of the mental processes engaged, or of the factors and influences addressed, until the therapist requests such awareness from Centrum.

In most instances, the therapist can employ ST as the sole treatment. However, in some situations it may be more effectively employed as an adjunct to other modes of treatment. If the patient demonstrates resistance to therapy in the use of other psychological interventions, an excursion into the process of ST may resolve the resistance and permit resumption of the original treatment. In any event, and regardless of the technique being employed in therapy, ST can be used as a means of systematic uncovering, of measuring progress in therapy, and possibly of testing attainment of the therapeutic goal.

Chapter III

The Process of Subliminal Therapy

Once the therapist has instructed the patient as to his or her role during the procedure of ST, the therapist guides the patient to begin direct, purposeful interactions with Centrum. Having defined the goal(s) to be addressed, and having established communication with Centrum, the sequence of questions and requests to Centrum follows a logical, decision-tree format. One version of this format is described by means of the flow charts detailed in Appendix A.

What the Clinician Must Know

Patients readily accommodate the concepts of ST. These concepts of subconscious functioning and conditioning are likely to be familiar to the patient before treatment begins, with only the concept of Centrum requiring real explanation. As the guide in the process, the clinician must have clear comprehension of the pragmatic elements of communicating with Centrum. These elements are addressed in following paragraphs.

Posing Questions to Centrum

At least in the beginning of the work, questions should be posed to Centrum in a direct way, as though you are speaking to a separate person who is sitting there. To an uninformed observer, this format might seem odd, if not incongruous; however, the patient will have no difficulty transitioning to this format of communication and will also probably begin to demonstrate the signs associated with the trance state of hypnosis. That is to say,

diaphragmatic breathing, eye roll, absence of volitional movement and flaccid muscle tone will likely become apparent during
the course of your interactions.

You should pose questions in a direct, concrete, non-ambiguous,
simplistic format, with no implied or double-meaning elements.
Consistently preface questions to Centrum with the name
'Centrum' to clarify that the question is addressed to Centrum,
as opposed to the conscious mind of the patient, thereby cuing
the patient to respond with the answers appearing on the chalkboard. *It is of essential importance that you phrase the questions
clearly*; subconscious interpretation of the question will be literal
and confusion will otherwise result. A fair guide: Phrase your
questions as though speaking to someone new to the English
language.

Examples:

> If you want to know how old the patient is, ask, *"Centrum,
> how old are you now?"* as opposed to *"Centrum, do you know
> how old you are?"*

> If you want to know whether or not Centrum knows how
> old the patient was at some previous time ask, *"Centrum, do
> you know how old you were at that time?"*

Make your questions logical in format and sequence. If a deviation into a related subject is necessary – deviating from the
logic of the decision tree as illustrated in Appendix A – inform
Centrum that you are deviating before asking the question.
Then, when returning to the decision tree is indicated, state
that fact before asking the next question. In other words, keep
Centrum informed about what you are doing as in the following
examples:

> *Centrum, do you believe you understand why you felt so depressed?*

> *Centrum, it is often true that when people are depressed they also
> feel anxious. Does any part of your mind now feel anxious?*

Centrum, we will address that anxiety after we complete the depression issue we are working on. Let's return now to the depression issue. Would it be okay for you to have conscious awareness of the cause of the depression?

While it is true that the usual responses from Centrum are expressed in the energy-conserving words, "Yes" and "No", there will be an occasional patient of high IQ whose Centrum will respond elaborately and orally. Such responses give rise to questions about whether or not they are conscious opinions, but when adequately reassured by the patient that they are, in fact, communications from Centrum, therapy proceeds even more efficiently.

Recognizing Responses That Were Presented As Coming From Centrum, But Are Expressions Of Conscious Opinion

The process of ST is guided by responses from Centrum. Therapeutic success demands that you detect responses from the patient that are instead expressions of conscious opinion, and that are presented to you as though being responses from Centrum. To continue the course of treatment guided by conscious responses is to guarantee failure in outcome. Yet, despite pointed emphasis on the *essential* importance of their reporting ONLY what is written on the chalkboard, patients will sometimes slip out of their role as observers, even without conscious intent to do so (see Chapter V for further expansion of this problem).

Fortunately, most responses of conscious opinion are easily detected. If the response is "It says ...," or "There's a Yes and a No," the answer is surely from Centrum. On the other hand, if the response is "I think so" or is more than a few words in length, odds are it is not from Centrum. If you have a question about any response, ask about it in a direct way such as *"Was that answer written on the chalkboard?"* or *"I remind you of the essential importance of your reporting to me ONLY what is written on the chalkboard. Was that answer written on your chalkboard?"*

On occasion, the patient may knowingly and consistently report conscious opinions in lieu of responses from Centrum, doing so in ways that raise suspicion in your mind as to their origin but that seem substantiated by responses to the questions you have posed. When this happens, I have found that the patient is usually doing their best, possibly disbelieving that Centrum will respond, or possibly unwilling to displease me by giving no report, yet not actually perceiving answers on the chalkboard. Frank, compassionate discussion usually reveals what is happening and repeating the instructions on the use of the chalkboard can usually facilitate return to therapy. The use of ideo-motor responses or another vehicle of communication may also solve the problem, allowing treatment to proceed. In many of these cases, after the patient has subjectively experienced the validity of the communications from Centrum by another means, they may then become able to use the chalkboard.

In my experience, only about 2 percent of treated patients have not been able to perceive and report communications from Centrum by one vehicle or another. In those rare cases when communication is not possible, I revert to hypnotic age regression techniques coupled with direct suggestion. If that is not fruitful, I use conventional, direct hypnotic suggestions as an option and combine them with cognitive work to clarify issues and to inspire the patient to consider things from another perspective.

Resistance

Resistance to change is a universal human experience; in general we like things to stay the same. However, when someone consciously desires a change that does not spontaneously happen, we must conclude that resistance originates from the subconscious domain. In the model of ST, we assume that a distinct part (or parts) holds opinions that are in disagreement with conscious opinion, causing the presenting problem to continue.

In applying ST, the clinician often finds evidence of subconscious resistance, usually during the early steps of application.

The most frequently encountered evidence becomes apparent when the chalkboard is suddenly not available to the patient; it disappears. Less frequently, 'fog' may obscure the chalkboard, there may be no response at all, or the chalkboard may be too far away to read. There may be misleading or nonsensical answers, or other indications of unwillingness to cooperate. The clinical skills of the therapist are challenged to persuade, bypass or overwhelm the resisting parts. Consider the following possibilities; if one is not effective, employ another:

- In speaking to the part, be persuasive. Acknowledge the part as being well-intended. Request the part to consider present life circumstances and the need for the desired change.

- Request the resisting part to listen as the patient verbalizes the reasons he/she desires the goal. This may seem awkward (having the patient talk to him/herself); however, it is often effective.

- Request that Centrum communicate with the part, that Centrum accomplish the task without your assistance. (Assume that Centrum hears you. You may be working in the blind, since you have no communications from Centrum, yet it is probable that Centrum can hear you.)

- Negotiate a trial period during which, and under some condition, the work can proceed. Propose this to the resisting part even though it feels like talking to the ether.

- Use another vehicle of communication such as an inner voice or ideo-motor responses.

- Attempt to overwhelm the resistance by authoritative voice tones, essentially commanding that the work be permitted to proceed.

I have included a more thorough discussion of resistance, and techniques for resolving resistance, in Chapter VI under *Subconscious Resistance to Change*.

Maintain the Focus of the Procedure on the Immediate Goal to be Achieved

One of the first tasks to accomplish is to assist the patient in defining the goals of the work. Once defined, prioritize them based primarily on the patient's sense of importance, yet with consideration for your clinical judgment. Once prioritized, address the goals individually, even if overlapping issues between them become apparent. If you achieve one goal in the course of identifying and resolving the causal issues of another goal, which will commonly happen, so much the better. For example, if having identified and resolved the causes of a headache, another problem, anxiety, ceases to exist.

It is not difficult to become derailed from a logical sequence of steps by a related issue that comes up. Yield not to temptation; stay focused on the original goal.

Initial Patient Preparation

Ensure patients understand that they provide the problem, the motivation to resolve the problem and the intellectual capacity to do so. The therapist teaches the patient 'how to' and guides the process.

The patient wants to know what to expect, and the therapist must so inform the patient for effective cooperation to be possible. The concepts of ST will be new to the patient and, just as small bites thoroughly chewed are more easily swallowed, so are the concepts of ST. The therapist should present them to the patient in small segments, explaining each in adequate detail and confirming understanding of each. Then, assuming the patient's understanding of the concepts of ST, the therapist should provide detailed instructions regarding the cooperation expected from the patient, which is to provide the communications link between Centrum and the therapist.

The Role of the Therapist

In general, clinicians with a psychodynamic perspective of life are trained to elicit historical information from the patient and then to assist the patient in re-evaluating or reframing that information. The point is, we are trained to be involved in all aspects of the process of therapy, including the content of the issues addressed. For example, in a typical session, we pay attention to the historical information presented by the patient, and we are sensitive to possible interactions and correlations unrecognized by the patient. When employing ST, the therapist is more divorced from content and may not be involved at all as long as Centrum is successfully accomplishing the work. In other words, the therapist may be blind to content. Actually, when employing ST, the therapist is encouraged to avoid involvement in the content of the material being addressed by the patient, and for this reason the transition from traditional techniques to employing ST may be challenging for some clinicians.

On the other hand, you will encounter situations in which the patient lacks the intellectual sophistication necessary to reframe or otherwise resolve the problem. Or, perhaps the patient may simply need pragmatic information upon which to base a decision, or may need advice. Under these conditions the therapist is called upon to contribute. Nevertheless, in almost all cases, the patient will benefit most from utilizing inner capabilities and perspectives whenever they suffice to resolve the problem. The therapist will be more effective if, in establishing rapport and educating the patient about ST, he leads the patient to the conviction of being in personal control and only being guided through the process by the therapist.

Moreover, the therapist should refrain from forming assumptions about probable causes of presenting problems. I have learned that I am seldom correct when I make such assumptions. It is better to be curious about what the cause will turn out to be, as an erroneous assumption on your part could result in misleading the patient. Initially, patients commonly believe they know why they have a given problem. They may come close, but (consciously) they never fully understand the cause–effect relationships involved and are consistently surprised when they comprehend those relationships.

As the therapist employing ST, your overall objective should be to teach the patient the skills necessary to accomplish desired change, and then to guide the patient to use those skills to accomplish their goal.

I endorse the teachings of Carl Rogers (1951); psychotherapy must be client centered if it is to be effective. We must show unconditional positive regard for the patient and, to the extent the patient perceives the therapist as critical, paradoxically the patient must defend the very position that is problematic, leading to a resistant patient. The patient's values, opinions and beliefs must be utilized. The therapist cannot know all of the issues to be considered, therefore the therapist's opinions have no place in the content of therapy. These principles apply with unique force when ST is employed.

'Be with' the patient, especially in the beginning. Be emotionally attuned to the patient. Be sensitively aware of the patient's situation and concerns, thereby establishing rapport. If the patient becomes emotionally labile while addressing a serious issue, be there as an anchor and intercede before things get out of hand. If appropriate, use touch to affirm your being there. Place your hand on the patient's hand or forearm and say words such as *"That was only a memory"* or *"You are here with me now, and you can feel the touch of my hand,"* thereby providing an anchor to present experience. You will establish trust by your being there, making it possible for the patient to go to the necessary mental place and to do the necessary work, even if some present trauma due to an abreaction should occur.

The Role of the Patient

Initially and on an ongoing basis, the patient consciously defines the direction of the work of therapy, doing so before treatment begins. The patient defines the goals, although perhaps with the assistance of the therapist in refining their expression. The patient provides the motivation to do the work, as well as the values and beliefs that guide the work. Having done so, and unless requested to express conscious opinion, the patient then cooperates passively in the process by maintaining sensitivity to the communications from Centrum, reporting those communications to the therapist.

Defining the Goal(s) of Therapy

Sometimes a patient presents just one goal, but usually there is more than one. The clinician's task is to assist the patient in defining, and often separating, the problem(s) presented. The goals will guide the solutions to the problems. See the case histories in Chapter V for illustrations of this principle.

The patient has often defined a general objective, such as "I want to be happy," but has not defined the specifics of how to achieve that objective; it is necessary to identify the specific barriers to being happy. The patient may not be consciously aware of the existence of the barriers and will not be aware of their identity, even if aware of their existence. In further illustration, if the patient presents with a sleeping problem, the goal might be defined in specific, affirmative terms such as "Eliminate the barriers to sleeping well" or "Postpone until later those thoughts that prevent sleep."

The Concept of Conditioning

It is no surprise to reasoning people that we are conditioned by the experiences we have. We were taught to believe what we believe. We have the skills, values and limitations we learned in the course of living. Of course, genetic factors, and perhaps spiritual factors as well, have direct impact on conditioning, but life experience is responsible for the conditioning that results in most presenting, psychological problems. In essence, we *learn* to feel good, or anxious, or depressed, or to experience asthma or irritable bowel syndrome. Moreover, we learn without being consciously aware that conditioning is taking place at the time it is taking place.

This being true, and recognizing that our conditioning changes as we learn different values, skills and contexts, it follows that we can resolve an undesired consequence of conditioning by reconditioning. The essential purpose of ST is to accomplish change by such reconditioning. In ST, the undesired conditioning is conceptualized as being represented by some part of the mind, with many other parts representing other conditioned elements. The first task is to identify the responsible part and then to recondition that part by educating the part about current reality, contrasting this with the reality of life when the part came into being.

Smooth muscle responds to conditioning via the autonomic nervous system, and many physical disorders and illnesses are directly caused by the action of smooth muscle under that control. Bronchial asthma, for example, is a potentially life-threatening illness that occurs when smooth muscles occlude the bronchial passageways in the lungs and throat. Irritable bowel syndrome is the consequence of the non-sequential action of smooth muscles in the stomach, coupled with the action of related glands that disrupt the digestive process. Tension and migraine headaches are caused by smooth muscles creating cranial pressure. The etiology of these disorders may thus be psychogenic and in my experience commonly are.

Since the action of smooth muscles is controlled subconsciously, it makes sense to treat psychogenic illnesses by correcting the subconscious process that is causing the problem. ST is the intervention of choice. By its use, the subconscious *causes* of the illness can be uncovered and resolved; the symptoms, or at least those symptoms that are psychogenic, then cease to exist.

Introducing the Concept of Subliminal Therapy to the Patient

As mentioned previously, the therapist can introduce the concept of ST to the patient by means other than lecture. However, even when the patient has prior information, such as from having read the introductory booklet (Yager, 1985), I still advise reviewing the concepts with the patient at the beginning of treatment. When the patient understands the concepts, the stage is set for the work of therapy. By discussion and gentle inquiry, ensure that the patient understands each of the following points:

- Our mental functioning is in part conscious, but takes place in much greater part without conscious awareness. For example, the exceedingly complex regulation of bodily functions necessary to maintain life, functions such as the regulation of the pattern of blood flow, glandular functioning, digestive processes and breathing, take place without conscious awareness.

- Conditioning from life experience determines our beliefs, values, skills and limitations. In greater part we learn constructive things, such as how to function effectively. Yet we also learn harmful things that cause problems. That conditioning must be changed to correct the problems. This is the task of psychotherapy.

- The subconscious domain of the mind consists, at least in large part, of the multitude of conditioned parts that developed during the course of living. Each part represents some learned value, skill or limitation, or may represent an influence that reinforces another influence from an earlier experience, be it positive or negative in nature.

- Our ability to consciously control our behavior is limited by subconscious conditioning; e.g., we might learn that we are helpless to control something.

- Some level of conflict will inevitably exist between the parts of our mind. For example, most of us wish something was different about ourselves, that we had some ability or that we didn't have a certain limit. When that conflict interferes with happiness, or when we recognize something is wrong, it is time to seek professional assistance.

* We all have a 'higher level of intelligence'. This higher intelligence is well-intentioned, supporting life's needs and maintaining order among the many parts of the subconscious mind. This higher intelligence has the ability to learn new things, to access memories and to communicate with other parts in the subconscious domain. I call this higher intelligence Centrum.

* Assuming willingness to do so, Centrum can accomplish the work of therapy in highly efficient ways, guided by the therapist, yet without the therapist being involved in the content of the work.

* The therapist must be able to communicate with Centrum in order to guide the process.

* Centrum is usually aware of present circumstances and so is aware of what the therapist is saying.

* The necessary additional element is a vehicle to receive communication *from* Centrum. The cooperation of the patient is required to supply that communication.

Instructing the Patient in Perceiving Communications from Centrum

Communication from Centrum can come only via the patient; however, it may come in different forms as described below. The most flexible and efficient means is visual, such as an imagined chalkboard or computer screen. Children often prefer an imagined computer screen, while adults usually find an imaginary chalkboard to be effective. Other patients sometimes choose from various forms of visual imagery such as a blank space. In all events, Centrum is requested to write on the medium, with the patient reporting to the therapist what has been written. The advantages of the chalkboard include being able to re-examine what is written, and the responses can be validated as coming from Centrum by questioning the form of the letters. Also, there is no limit to the length or structure of the responses, even though they will usually be brief.

Alternate Means of Perceiving Communications from Centrum

In a few cases, visual communications from Centrum do not seem possible and the patient must employ other vehicles. Such alternate means of perceiving communications include the following:

An inner voice may be perceived by the patient. This option has the advantage of not being restricted to "Yes" and "No" answers, as in some of the other approaches; however, the responses are only fleeting, i.e., they cannot be re-examined by the patient and so validity cannot be acquired easily.

Ideo-motor responses via finger signals may be employed. As taught by LeCron (1965) and Ewin (2006), such responses are an option for all but the most resistant patient. In this approach, the patient is asked to place his open, dominant hand, with fingers extended and palm down, on the arm of the chair, on his thigh or, preferably, on his stomach. Coded meanings are then assigned to the fingers, usually with the index finger representing "Yes," the middle finger meaning "No," the little finger meaning "I don't know" and the thumb meaning "I don't want to answer." As instructed by the therapist, the correct answer is to be indicated by Centrum causing the appropriate finger to rise. The therapist instructs the patient to avoid consciously lifting or interfering with the lifting of the fingers, and Centrum is asked to indicate understanding of the coded meanings by causing the "Yes" finger to rise. Assuming the requested response is given, the sequence of treatment begins.

Since responses from Centrum are limited to a Yes/No option, the questions posed must be phrased such that answers in this format are sensible. Treatment, therefore, becomes more ponderous and time consuming with this method.

Chevreul's pendulum can be used. The pendulum can be a necklace, watch and chain or any other object suspended by a string or chain. The patient holds the pendulum by the thumb and one finger suspended over a drawing that shows four different directions of swing, corresponding to "Yes," "No," "I don't know" and "I don't want to answer." This drawing is depicted in Figure 1.

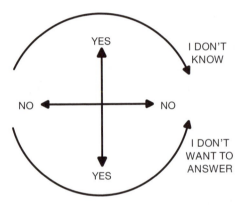

Figure 1 – Suggested coded meaning for the pendulum

Centrum is then requested to communicate by causing the pendulum to swing in the appropriate direction, and the patient is cautioned not to consciously intervene in any way, neither causing nor impeding its swing. This technique seems to be the most sensitive of all techniques. Responses can be elicited without benefit of trance, and essentially everyone can experience such responses, although more time is required to set the stage and there are greater response times for the answers.

Ouija boards can be employed effectively since responses with this method are not limited to a Yes/No option. Responses, however, are much more time consuming than by means of a chalkboard.

Automatic writing is another option. The patient is equipped with paper and pencil, placed in the position to write, with pencil poised above the paper. Centrum is requested to take control of the pencil and write the answers on the paper. Trance may be necessary for the technique to be effective; however, all advantages of the chalkboard are potentially present except time efficiency; automatic writing responses are consistently slow in execution.

A computer keyboard and monitor is an interesting option. I have presented it last in this series only because the necessary equipment is not typically available in the psychotherapy setting. Centrum is requested to type the answers, with the result that this approach is more time efficient than the automatic writing option and retains most of the advantages of the chalkboard.

To simplify the instructions, I start by asking the patient to visualize a chalkboard. If that proves difficult, I suggest the use of a television or computer screen. If that response is not fulfilled, I will switch to another of the possible means of response. All else failing, I will finally resort to the use of a pendulum last, primarily because of the excessive time required for the responses to occur.

Assuming the patient is able to visualize a chalkboard, which is true in a high percentage of cases, I ask Centrum to indicate willingness to communicate by this means by writing the word "Yes" on the chalkboard. I ask the patient to advise me when that word appears. When the patient reports the "Yes" response, I will typically guide him/her to validate the response by the challenge: *"You might very reasonably say to me that you can imagine a chalkboard with "Yes" or "No" or anything else on it, and therefore wonder how you can tell if the answer came from Centrum."* I will acknowledge the validity of the question and point out: *"You can, of course, do what you wish consciously, yet, if Centrum writes the word, it is probable that you will not be able to erase it."* I will then invite the patient to try to erase the word, and only rarely will the patient be able to do so. The experience of being unable to erase the word is usually satisfying to the patient, and the work can proceed without the distraction of wondering about the responses. If further validation is needed, I will request that Centrum replace the word "Yes" with a different word, a word that Centrum is requested to select, a word that will surprise the patient, thereby validating the response.

In the event that responses from Centrum are perceived by means other than the chalkboard, I pursue validation of those responses by means similar to the above but adapted to the vehicle of communication available. In any event, validation of the reality of communication from Centrum is of value to both patient and therapist.

Teenagers consistently find the phenomenon of communicating with their higher intelligence to be fascinating and challenging. Working through barriers to performance with this group is fun in the most beneficial way; they work so rapidly you will be challenged to keep up with them.

The 'Guiding Rule'

The initial task of ST consists of setting the stage for actual treatment to begin. The goal of therapy must be defined, the patient must be educated about the concepts of ST and the process to be engaged and communications with Centrum must be established. Finally, the therapist should obtain commitment from the patient to comply with the 'Guiding Rule' as expressed in the following example of communication to the patient:

> *I'd like to set up a guiding rule for us to use as we work together. To avoid confusion about whether I am communicating with Centrum, or whether I am communicating with you consciously, I propose the following rule: Any time I preface a question with the name "Centrum", the next word I hope to hear from you will be the words that are written on the chalkboard, as opposed to what you might think should be written there. I cannot see your chalkboard, and if you fill in a blank or change an answer, we will go down the wrong road, wasting my time and your money.*

Chapter IV

Applying Subliminal Therapy

To begin this phase, the therapist instructs the patient as to his or her role in the process of ST and then begins direct, purposeful interactions with Centrum. Having defined the goal to be addressed, and having established communications with Centrum, the sequence of questions and requests to Centrum follow a logical, decision-tree format. This format is described best by means of the flow charts detailed in Appendix A; however, the following description may aid in learning the process.

Introductory Questions

As a part of the required stage-setting, the therapist should pose a series of questions to Centrum. These questions ensure that Centrum is communicating in an acceptable manner, is capable of doing the required work and is willing to do the work. The following questions are suggested:

- *"Centrum, are you aware of your conscious concern about this problem?"*
  Ultimately, an affirmative answer is essential and explanations must be provided to Centrum by the therapist or by the patient to the extent that Centrum is aware of the problem. If the answer is negative, after requesting that Centrum listen, I will typically ask the patient to verbalize his or her concern. This accomplished, I will repeat the key question and continue explaining until an affirmative response is forthcoming.

- *"Centrum, are you willing to cooperate, to do some work as I guide you and teach you how, to eliminate the compulsion to wash your hands?"*

  An affirmative response is obtained in the great majority of cases; however, if not obtained, the therapist must explore the reason for the refusal and persuade Centrum to cooperate.

- *"Centrum, do you have the ability to look at memories of events that have happened in the past?*

  If an affirmative response is not obtained, ask Centrum if there is a memory of what was eaten for breakfast today. The answer will almost certainly be "Yes" and the therapist can ask other questions, reaching further and further back in time. When such memories are evident, point out that Centrum *can* access memories and move on to the next question.

- *"Centrum, do you have the ability to communicate with other parts of the mind?"*

  An affirmative response can usually be expected, but if not expressed, you, as the therapist, can remind Centrum that communication is taking place here and now, that communication need not be by means of words and that you believe Centrum can actually establish such communications. *"Centrum, be aware that you are already communicating."*

The Flow Charts

Introduction to the Flow Charts

The flow charts in Appendix A are intended as aids in learning to apply ST. The steps presented are the steps I typically take, based on my thirty-five years of experience with ST. These steps are not necessarily the best selection in terms of content, or in terms of order of presentation; they are, rather, my personal, biased view of the preferred path to take. Yours may be better, yet I suggest you begin learning ST with mine.

Following the flow charts in Appendix A, I offer suggested words for use in the steps of the flow charts. As the clinician, you will ultimately employ phrasing and expressions that are personally comfortable and natural for you to use. It is the meaning and flow that must be communicated. This is as it should be. Some clinicians will adhere to my words, and that's okay too, as they are good words and have proven to be effective. Moreover, not all possible paths of treatment are covered by the flow charts, yet they will prove sufficient in most cases. Your knowledge and skills as a clinician will be required to devise alternate paths in other cases.

Instructions for Using the Flow Charts

These charts are intended for instructional purposes; they do not cover all possible courses treatment might take. They are adequate for many cases, but as many more will deviate to the extent of requiring innovation and creative thought on your part as the clinician.

As you learn to use ST, you may find better sequences to use, and you are encouraged to use what works for you; nevertheless, the sequence provided is a tool to use in developing your skills.

Practice is of course essential. Read the content until you know what the next words are apt to be. If you comprehend the logic of the flow of the process, you will find that it flows for you.

Your patient will likely slip into trance during the instructions for communicating with Centrum. Therefore, you will not be observed as you read the content suggested for the flow charts. It will be important that you read in your own, natural voice, rather than a voice that reveals you are reading; this is easily achieved through minimal practice. Trust that the patient is involved in his or her own thoughts and experiences and will not be paying critical attention to your performance. Speak clearly and with confidence; all else will follow as you would wish.

Applications of Subliminal Therapy

Treating Pain with Subliminal Therapy

Albert Schweitzer once called pain "a more terrible lord of mankind than even death itself." Even so, pain is essential to life; we simply could not live without it. We would behave in self-destructive ways without being aware that we were doing so. Yet, pain can also be dysfunctional, creating unnecessary distress. The latter condition is addressed here.

Some Rules about Pain

- Pain is about perception, and perception can be altered with hypnosis.
- Pain is always real to the person in pain.
- Pain always has a purpose.
- Chronic pain always has a subconscious purpose.
- Physical pain can be caused either by physical or emotional trauma.

The Purpose of Pain

Pain is the mind's way of getting attention; it is essentially a protective mechanism. When pain happens, it is a message to do something – change the situation, let go of that hot dish, see a doctor, do something! Then, having done all that you know to do, the pain no longer has a purpose and it becomes possible not to perceive it, even when it has organic origin. This may sound simplistic; however, it is reality.

When pain persists unnecessarily, it is because we have learned to continue to perceive it. Perhaps we have subconsciously learned to *expect* it to continue, or we have subconsciously become aware that the pain has value (e.g., it gets attention or permits us to avoid a situation). Note that I said 'subconsciously', as we may not be consciously aware that we are learning a lesson. If a dog bites a child, the child will learn to fear dogs. The child is not aware that he is learning to fear dogs; it happens without conscious awareness. In the same way, we may learn to associate pain with other things, doing so without conscious awareness. As examples, we might learn that the presence of pain means we are still alive, or that pain motivates us to do something.

Especially in the case of chronic pain, whether of physical or mental origin, the actual subconscious purpose of the pain is rarely recognized consciously, and pain can persist long after the original purpose of the pain ceases to exist. In such a situation, the pain is maintained by subconscious influence, for reasons that were real and valid in the past – when the pain began – but are no longer real or valid. When both conscious and subconscious domains recognize that the pain no longer has valid purpose, either direct hypnotic suggestions or an analytic hypnotic approach such as ST can be employed to relieve the suffering. However, conscious desire alone is not sufficient for relief; there must be an absence of subconscious resistance from parts that believe relieving the pain would be ill-advised.

Treating Pain by Hypnotic Techniques

Our minds have the ability to simply not perceive pain. This ability is accessible via hypnosis for most people and is used for surgical anesthesia in appropriate situations. However, to use this capacity without consideration of the purpose of the pain is clearly contra-indicated, since to do so might endanger the person, as might happen if the pain is from an impending appendix rupture. Either direct or indirect hypnotic suggestions may relieve pain, at least temporarily. However, the use of hypnotic techniques to identify and resolve the subconscious purpose(s) of the pain will usually be required to provide lasting relief. Subliminal Therapy is the treatment of choice for this task: resolve the purpose of the pain and the pain can then be relieved.

On the other hand, when the hypnotic trance state is employed for direct and/or indirect suggestions for relief, relief *can* be complete. For example, in emergent situations, when the patient's attention is focused on the attending physician (an example of hypnotic trance without formal induction), comments and suggestions by that physician can have a profound and long-lasting effect, either for good or for ill.

Some degree of relief from pain can be obtained by altering perception via other means, taking steps that can be understood as hypnotic, yet are not obviously hypnotic. For example, early in my treatment of pain, I may point out that *"If a large and ferocious dog were to come through that door right now, clearly about to attack you, you would not at that moment be aware of anything except the presence of the dog; you would be unaware of your pain. You would be experiencing the ability of your mind to direct your conscious attention away from the pain. This is an illustration of hypnotic phenomena, and as we work together I will be teaching you how to utilize hypnotic phenomena to mitigate the pain you have been experiencing."* Note that I have not promised to *eliminate* the pain, only to mitigate it. In some cases it may be possible to entirely eliminate the pain, and if so it should be done; however, some level of discomfort, in some situations, may be desirable for some purpose, whether the purpose is identified consciously or not.

In a few situations, the treatment can be to teach the patient to perceive the pain in a different way; perhaps a brief tickle, itch or other sensation, or even a perceived but non-existent odor would serve to satisfy the unconscious need. This situation might apply where the pain has a valued, consciously identified purpose, such as a means to avoid some situation, and it is subconsciously okay not to suffer from it.

We are talented at taking advantage of whatever life offers; we derive benefit where none is at first apparent (e.g., pain as a way of getting attention or sympathy, often called secondary gain). These benefits are seldom recognized consciously and can become the basis for maintaining the pain. To achieve relief, the benefits must be identified and considered in the light of current, more objective knowledge. Then, assuming the conclusion is reached that the benefit is no longer present, or that it is not worth the penalty (the pain), subconscious conditioning can be reversed and the pain relieved. However, until all such subconscious benefits or purposes have been identified and resolved, direct hypnotic suggestion will likely provide only short-term relief.

Whether the pain is caused emotionally or physically, treatment should begin the same way. First, educate the patient about subconscious involvement in pain, then explore that involvement. Since the patient has no conscious awareness of that involvement, treatment must address the subconscious domain directly, and all subconscious influence that might prolong the pain must be resolved. Again, employing Subliminal Therapy is the most effective and most efficient way to do this.

Some Classes of Pain

Acute pain. Acute pain is defined as pain having recent origin. Examples include a physical injury such as a broken arm, or an emotional shock such as losing something or someone of esteemed value. Even grief can cause muscles to cramp, resulting in pain. Since acute pain usually does not allow time to incorporate subconscious, secondary benefits from the pain, searching for subconscious influence is usually not necessary and direct hypnotic suggestions are apt to be effective, both for immediate and longer-term relief.

Chronic pain. Chronic pain is defined as ongoing pain, or at least pain with few periods of respite. Typical examples include the pain associated with arthritis and spinal injury. These types of pain can be responsibly managed with hypnotic techniques, but probably only after medical treatment that satisfies the patient that everything known has been done. As in acute pain, immediate relief can probably be obtained by direct or indirect hypnotic suggestion; however, prolonged relief will most likely require an analytic approach such as Subliminal Therapy.

Severe pain. Either physical or psychological causes can be at the root of severe pain, and both can be alleviated with hypnotic techniques. This is true because, regardless of the cause and regardless of the severity, pain is always about perception. An advantage of hypnosis in dealing with severe pain is that a change in perception – disassociation – can be experienced more easily. Since disassociation is alteration of perception, and pain is about perception, the pain can be disassociated.

Episodic pain. Examples of episodic pain are migraine and tension headaches. The fact that the pain is episodic makes it unlikely that it has physical cause. For example, organically caused pain from a brain tumor does not present episodically, nor does the pain associated with cancer, although it can vary over time. Nevertheless, if pain ceases between episodes, it is most likely psychogenic. The subconscious purpose of episodic pain, just like other classes of pain, must be identified and resolved before effective, lasting relief can occur. In the meantime, direct hypnotic suggestion may provide significant temporary relief, and the use of self-hypnosis can also be of value in masking non-functional pain.

Phantom pain. The most common example of this class of pain is phantom limb pain. Here, pain is perceived to emanate from a location that no longer physically exists, for example, from an amputated leg. However, there are other cases in which pain is reported to be experienced outside the body, in some other phantom location, as though it has been disassociated. Often, the abrupt cessation of pain in response to direct hypnotic suggestion is sufficient to bring about permanent relief; however, long-term relief can be better assured by resolving related subconscious beliefs that might cause it to continue. For example, if the patient has unconsciously learned that pain has the benefit of getting love, it is apt to continue (in spite of the opposing conscious, rational opinion of the patient) until that subconscious belief has been identified and resolved.

Emotional pain. We speak of emotional pain in the same framework as physical pain, and it can evolve into actual physical pain through the action of smooth muscles as they react to the emotion. Protracted anger can result in stomach pain, for example. Also, verbal expressions of emotional pain parallel those of physical pain, perhaps constituting an unrecognized suggestion to experience physical pain.

Possible Subconscious Causes of Pain

Subconsciously inspired self-punishment is often involved in causing and sustaining pain; some long-forgotten unfortunate act, even though it is now understandable, can cause such self-punishing behavior. Moreover, it seems true that relief from *emotional* pain can often be achieved by experiencing *physical* pain. There might be a subconscious belief that pain is deserved, inevitable or unavoidable.

The pain could be a way to stay awake or to avoid awareness of something else. In short, any imaginable reason could be the cause of continued pain, and our imaginations know no limits. As stated above, the task of relieving subconsciously inspired pain *must* include identifying and resolving all subconscious basis for the pain.

We learn not to do that which causes pain; we learn to protect ourselves. This is good, yet, if what we learn is appropriate for only that situation, at that time – and not for other situations at other times – we may have learned a dysfunction. For example, in a time of trauma, with adrenalin flowing, a person might learn to associate pain with knowing they are still alive (for reasons not understood, adrenalin cements memories). Whatever the lesson, it had great importance in the original situation and yet would be irrelevant and dysfunctional if protracted over time.

With the use of Subliminal Therapy, a significant number of my patients have succeeded in relieving severe, chronic pain that resulted from injuries and surgeries experienced years ago, including injuries that have required morphine patches for relief until treated by Subliminal Therapy.

Using Subliminal Therapy to Treat Chronic Pain

I recommend the following steps be taken:

1. Educate the patient about pain and its psychic aspects, possibly by reading this chapter.

2. Teach the patient the skill of self-hypnosis and encourage practice.

3. Assuming the patient is responsive to hypnotic suggestions, such as a pleasant early memory or the numbing of a hand, follow such an episode by guiding the patient to experience at least some generalized relief from the presenting pain, *"Now, while you are experiencing trance."* Then, whether or not the patient has been hypnotically responsive, proceed with the protocol of Subliminal Therapy.

4. Guide Centrum to identify and resolve all subconscious influences that might cause or exacerbate the pain.

5. Guide Centrum to provide at least some immediate relief from any current pain, and request that Centrum continue to maintain that relief at the level of intensity Centrum deems appropriate.

6. Guide Centrum to inform all parts of the mind of the work just accomplished, so that uniform cooperation becomes possible in maintaining relief.

7. Request that Centrum provide conscious understanding of the influences just resolved, and discuss those influences with the patient to the extent necessary for the patient to clearly understand how each influence had contributed to the pain.

Treating PTSD with Subliminal Therapy

Posttraumatic stress disorder has become widely recognized, especially with respect to returning veterans; however, the diagnosis applies in a wide variety of settings. Although not meeting the specific criteria of PTSD, the consequence of traumatic experience can manifest as sexual dysfunction, general anxiety, depression, phobias, compulsion, obsessions and many other presenting problems, all without being recognized or diagnosed as a posttraumatic disorder. Posttraumatic effects are the most common basis for problems in my practice.

As I comprehend PTSD, it is explained by the theory of ST: One or more parts of the patient's mind, parts that were created at the time of the trauma, continue to believe the trauma is happening *now* and are reacting accordingly. That being said, it follows that treatment by ST would be the treatment of choice, and my experience in the treatment of the disorder affirms that statement.

While it is true that the number of treated PTSD patients is small, it is also true that trauma is the common denominator of the genesis of most of the many cases I have documented. It is not surprising that I achieved high rates of success.

Treating Migraine and Tension Headaches with Subliminal Therapy

Migraine and tension headaches are, regardless of assigned classification, the immediate, physiological consequence of cranial pressure. The pressure can be caused by infection, a tumor, or it can be generated by the action of smooth muscle. In the case of a tumor, the presentation of a headache probably will be constant and unrelenting. In the case of smooth muscle action, the presentation will probably be irregular and influenced by identifiable events, although this simple guide can be misleading and medical consultation is indicated.

The model of ST assumes the existence of subconscious influence, activating smooth muscle as the cause of non-organically based headaches, an assumption that has been validated by their successful elimination by ST. By far the greatest number of all headaches are psychogenic, and as such can be treated psychologically.

The treatment protocol for headaches is the same as for the many other psychogenic problems: Identify and resolve the causal influences.

Treating Depression and Anxiety with Subliminal Therapy

Depression and anxiety are – quite simply – the consequence of life experience. They do not stand as isolated problems. They are a re-experience of earlier experiences and represent the continuing influence of past experiences.

Depression and anxiety are the two most common mental health problems being treated in this country. Although there are many proposed treatments, by far the most commonly employed is the use of psychotropic medication. Yet, according to Robert Whitaker in his wonderful book, *Anatomy of an Epidemic* (2010), the consequence of using currently available psychotropic medications is disastrous in the long term, even though often beneficial in the short term.

Depression and anxiety are commonly thought of, and treated, as though they are stand-alone disorders. This model is based on the concept of their resulting from a chemical imbalance in the brain; however, such is not the case. They are the after-effect, the consequence, of events in life, and the much-researched and publicized chemical imbalance in the brain is a *consequence*, not the *cause* of the disorder. Therefore, ST is appropriate and effective as a treatment.

Treating Addictions with Subliminal Therapy

We speak of being addicted to street drugs and cigarettes, and we express concern about becoming addicted to medications. We also speak of being addicted to a behavior such as gambling, and of being addicted to another person. These are, in fact, legitimate statements in that they refer to obsessions over which we may have little or no control.

In the physiological sense of addiction, we speak in terms of withdrawal and tolerance, yet those reactions are, themselves, mental perceptions of physical processes. In other words, *all* addictions embrace mental disorders, and unless the causal mental issues are resolved, control of the addiction will be difficult at best. This is not to deny the physical component, which can even be life-threatening and demands medical management. However, with abstinence, the physical (chemical) components of the addiction yield their power over time. In the case of tobacco smoke, it is in the order of a week; in the case of heroin, it is months to years in duration.

To date, with the exception of smoking cessation cases, I have had only minimal experience in treating chemical addictions with ST, yet those cases I have treated affirm that a major, if not *the* major, component of these addictions is the mental component. This mental component is the result of conditioning by life experiences, just like the many other problems discussed in this book, and as such it can be corrected. Here again, ST is the treatment of choice for correction.

In the case of chemical addictions, in addition to the usual sequence of ST treatment employed for other problems, the use of direct hypnotic suggestions for the relief of withdrawal discomfort can be valuable, especially when reinforced by the influence of Centrum. Additionally, direct suggestion can accelerate the rate of the withdrawal process.

A highly important aspect of your treatment should be that you follow the patient for at least the duration of the metabolism and elimination of the addicting chemical from the body. Not to do so invites relapse as other issues surface, issues that can be resolved with ST at each following visit.

Treating Vaginismus with Subliminal Therapy

Vaginismus is a frequently encountered problem that is often regarded as a physical, sexual problem. Vaginismus involves the contraction of the muscles at the entrance to the vaginal canal to occlude that passageway, thus preventing sexual intercourse. It is a classic example of psychic influence manifesting directly as a physical problem.

In my experience, vaginismus is a physical defense to unwanted penetration. It is psychogenic and should be treated as being psychogenic. The Masters and Johnson treatment protocol of the 1960s has been the standard treatment, effective in many cases in spite of its disadvantages. This treatment protocol involves progressive, forced enlargement of the vaginal opening and it is an unnecessary, painful and offensive approach that should be relegated to the archives of medicine along with blood-letting.

Treatment of vaginismus by Subliminal Therapy is simple and direct, avoiding the personal trauma of physical invasion. The reaction of the vaginal muscles that resist penetration is prompted by subconscious defense against some earlier violation. Uncovering and reframing that prior experience(s), most effectively accomplished by using Subliminal Therapy, will resolve the problem gently and effectively. This has been my experience in well over thirty cases over the past forty years and I do not recall a single failure. On the other hand, I do recall a number of cases of unsuccessful treatment by the Masters and Johnson progressive dilation approach that were subsequently resolved by Subliminal Therapy, and that were reported to me in terms that were not flattering to the medical profession.

Vaginismus, like gastro-intestinal issues, asthma and many other problems that manifest physically, can be psychogenic. Resolve the *cause* and the problem goes away, not just temporarily, it goes away, period.

Weight Management and Subliminal Therapy

Of all the problems treated by Subliminal Therapy, weight control is by far the most difficult to relieve. Once results are achieved, however, the transformation is dramatic, because the change encompasses not just reduction in weight, but improvements in personality, self-image and attitude as well.

Yet, in spite of modest success in controlling weight by Subliminal Therapy in the experience of the author, the road to completion can be longer than expected, and can be bumpy.

The essential causes of weight problems are either compulsive eating or an unconscious mandate to be heavy. When the cause is resolved, loss of weight becomes possible with less trauma and, unlike the typical cyclic pattern in which weight is regained, the loss is maintained.

The Benefits

For a fortunate few, the benefits of using Subliminal Therapy for control of weight seem immediate; for most, however, the benefits accrue gradually, even subtly, as changes in character take place. Along with awareness of effortless behavior change, the patient may notice in retrospect that there is no longer a desire for a particular food, or they may find they are eating less, or drinking less of an inappropriate beverage than before. The rate of change is not predictable, and in any event is not likely to be as rapid as might be wished, but once achieved the new pattern of eating behavior will have become a lasting aspect of the patient's nature, just as the previous pattern had been an aspect of previous nature.

The How

Every experience in life has an effect on us. The effects may be minuscule or dramatic, but even if minuscule, if they are many and related, the accumulated influence can be significant. Achieving control of eating behavior requires that each of those learned influences (those that are causing the excess weight) must be identified and resolved. Since, in the case of eating behaviors, conditioned associations between eating and other good things begin at birth or before, the total number of such associations is many-fold. They are not consciously recognized and so cannot be addressed consciously. This is where the advantages of Subliminal Therapy manifest as the most efficient and effective way to identify, and then to resolve, those influences. When the psychological barriers to being thin – or to controlled eating, as the case may be – have been set aside, the rate and specific procedure for loss of weight can be accelerated by any number of different programs.

Treatment

The treatment program for weight control using Subliminal Therapy will follow a predictable pattern. First, there will be an initial session of history-taking, evaluation and instruction. This will be followed by a series of sessions, occurring as frequently as possible, during which the bulk of influences that are causing the weight-producing behaviors will be identified and resolved. When this phase has been completed, and it is not possible to determine in advance when that will happen, the sessions will occur progressively less frequently and the benefits can be expected to have progressive impact.

No Guarantee

It is not possible to warrant or predict the total number of treatment sessions that may be required in a given case; they may be few or they may be many in number, depending upon the patient's life history. I have seen success in as few as seven total sessions, or in as many as forty. It can, however, be said with certainty that success in every case requires advanced, conscious commitment to complete the number of sessions required.

Effective treatment of these various disorders is, as with so many other disorders, best accomplished by uncovering and resolving the underlying psychological cause of the problem. This is, of course, a core theme of Subliminal Therapy, and the sequence of steps required is the same as for other disorders.

Chapter V

Case Illustrations

The following pages contain annotated transcriptions of various cases I have selected from my practice. A few of the cases are presented in full context; however, most are excerpted from the case histories to illustrate particular points. Names have been changed to avoid recognition and other demographic data are only approximately accurate. As a clinician learning Subliminal Therapy, you are encouraged to read these case histories in detail; a cursory review will not suffice to learn the nuances of the application of this technique.

The following details of font and capitalization apply in all of the cases as a way to understand "who" is communicating information.

Clinician speaking	Serif, Normal
Patient speaking	Serif, *Italic*
CENTRUM SPEAKING	Serif, CAPITALIZED
Another person speaking	Sans serif, Normal

Pat – A Case of Smoking Cessation

I have placed this case first in this chapter because of its uncomplicated, picture-perfect flow of the process of Subliminal Therapy and to present it almost in its entirety.

Pat was a 52-year-old Caucasian male who presented for smoking cessation. He had been smoking for thirty years at the rate of one pack per day. His wife did not smoke and he was under considerable family pressure to stop. Pat stated he enjoyed smoking to the extent that he considered it worth the financial cost, but not the price paid in family discomfort.

Pat was seen on three occasions. The first was an initial interview during which his history was taken, he was taught self-hypnosis as a personal skill and he was guided to compare his own lists of his reasons to stop smoking with his reasons to continue to smoke. He concluded without reservation that he truly desired to stop smoking. He was given the introductory book, *Subliminal Therapy: Utilizing the Unconscious Mind* (Yager, 1985), and was instructed to read the book before our next session. The following narration begins the second session, at which point he had read the book.

SECOND SESSION

Now, Pat, you might very reasonably point out that you can imagine a chalkboard with "yes" on it, or "no" on it, or whatever you want on it. How can you know if Centrum wrote that word on the chalkboard? At least in part, the answer is that if Centrum wrote the word on the chalkboard, in all probability you will find that you will not be able to erase it. Is the word "yes" still there on your chalkboard? *Yes.*

Good, then I invite you to try to erase it … Is it still there? *Yes.*

Centrum, please erase the word "yes" and replace it with a different word. This time, Centrum, I ask that you select a word that will surprise you consciously, some word that you will know you didn't consciously think up and write it on the chalkboard. Pat, let me know when that word appears and, if you are willing, tell me what the word is. *Thought.* Are you convinced you did not think that word up and put it there, that it is in fact a word that surprises you? *I don't know where that came from.*

Pat, that little exercise was not part of the work on your goals; it was only to show you that something different is working here. Now, I want to set up a 'Guiding Rule' for our use as we do this work. Anytime I preface a question, or request, with the name "Centrum," the

The application of Subliminal Therapy can be highly effective even without the patient believing in its validity. Nevertheless, the process will flow smoothly and with fewer snags if the patient can be made subjectively aware of the differences in his own perception as Centrum communicates.

The most frequently encountered problem in employing Subliminal Therapy is the substitution of *(continued)*

56

next thing I hope to hear from you will be the words Centrum writes on the chalkboard. You see, I can't see your chalkboard. I must assume what you tell me is in fact communication from Centrum. And any time you fill in a blank, or change an answer, perhaps because you don't consciously agree with it, at that moment we take off on an unproductive tangent and start wasting time. This work, you see, requires some mental discipline on your part. The chalkboard becomes a way to differentiate between your conscious opinions and the communications from Centrum. Bear in mind that your conscious opinion has not led you to the goal you seek; it's now time to do something different, and that difference is taking advantage of the abilities offered by Centrum. It's a very unusual thing to say to a patient, but when we are using Subliminal Therapy, I don't care what you think consciously; just tell me what Centrum writes on the chalkboard. Do you think you can do that? *Yes, I can.*

Good. Now we will begin the work you came to do.

Centrum, are you aware of your conscious concern about your smoking behavior? YES

Centrum, are you willing to cooperate, to do some work, as I guide you and teach you how, with the objective of eliminating that smoking behavior? YES, VERY MUCH

Centrum, just to be sure we are on common footing, I need to ask a couple of questions. Do you have the ability to remember things that happened in your past? That is, do you have the ability to access memories of events that have taken place? YES

Centrum, I will be asking that you identify different parts of your mind in preparation for communicating with them in the course of doing this work. Do you have the ability to communicate with different parts of your mind? YES

conscious opinion in lieu of communication from Centrum. It therefore becomes very important to stress the importance of consistently responding with the answers as they appear on the chalkboard. The Guiding Rule is one way to do so.

From this point forward, be sensitive to the words and the manner in which the words are expressed, as they are reported as coming from Centrum. In your practice, if you suspect a conscious response, question its source.

Centrum I believe you have abilities I don't even know how to talk about, and I now ask that you use those abilities, whatever they may be, to conduct an investigation into the cause of your smoking behavior. I ask that you review memories of those events in which you learned to smoke, and to communicate with other parts of your mind that may be involved in any way. It is the objective at this point, Centrum, for you to understand how, why, when and where you learned to smoke. In accomplishing this task, it's okay for you to work either with or without conscious awareness, as you deem appropriate. Centrum, is my request clear to you? YES

Then Centrum, please accomplish that request to the limit of your ability and let me know when you have completed the task, to the limit of your ability, by writing the word "complete" on the chalkboard. COMPLETE

Centrum, do you believe you understand why and how you learned to smoke? YES

Centrum, please identify that part, or parts, that came into existence in that situation, and that are still causing you to smoke. Is my request clear to you, Centrum? YES Then Centrum, please identify however many parts there are and let me know when you have completed the task by the word "complete" on the chalkboard. COMPLETE Centrum, did you identify one or more such parts? YES Centrum, how many such parts did you identify? FOUR Centrum, are you in communication with all four of those parts? YES

Centrum, please select one of those parts, perhaps the first part to come into existence, and communicate with that part in this way: First, listen to the part. Learn from the part what you need to know to be able to educate the part about present life situation, needs, values, etc. Centrum, that part is well-intended, but has been stuck back there in that time when it came

58

into existence, using its influence on the basis of what it understood when it came into existence. The problem is that what it understands is based on what was true when it came into existence, understanding that is no longer valid. Your task, Centrum, is to educate that part about your present reality, present life situation, needs and values. Persuade that part to your way of thinking so that it can support your present goal and wishes. Centrum, is my request clear to you? YES Then please Centrum, accomplish that task to the limit of your ability and let me know when you have done so by writing the word "complete" once again. COMPLETE Centrum, were you successful? Is that part now willing to support your conscious goal? YES

Centrum, please select a second of the four parts and repeat the same procedure you just employed. First, listen to the part, learn what you need to know, and then educate the part about present reality. Centrum, let me know by the word "complete" when you have completed the task. COMPLETE Centrum, were you successful? YES

Centrum, please repeat the same protocol you just used with each of the remaining parts, one at a time, each in its turn. First listen, then educate, and let me know by the word "complete" when you have completed the task. COMPLETE Centrum, were you successful in persuading both of those two parts to your way of thinking? YES

Centrum, it is very often true that when one influence has been identified and resolved, it then becomes possible, and perhaps **only** then, to identify another part, another influence that might cause the smoking behavior to continue. Please search into the far reaches of your mind to identify any part of your mind that, for any reason whatsoever, might cause you to continue smoking. Let me know by the word "complete" when you have done so. COMPLETE Centrum,

did you identify any remaining parts of your mind?
NO

Centrum, do you already have full conscious awareness and understanding of the work you just did,
including related memories and understanding of
how those events have impacted your life? YES

Very good work! Thank you, Centrum. Pat, does that
information make sense to you? Do you now consciously understand how and why you learned to
smoke? *Yes*

Then tell me, Pat, what are the four issues Centrum
just resolved?

*They were stress, relaxation, pleasure and sociability. I got
memories too.*

Pat, is there any reason, any benefit whatsoever, is
there any payoff in any form that would justify your
continuing to smoke for any of those four reasons?
No, there isn't.

Pat, the test of completeness of this work is in the real
world. As far as we know now, the work is complete,
meaning that you are now an ex-smoker. However,
there may yet be some part of your mind hiding over
there in the corner, saying something like, "You just
wait and see," some part that you have not yet identified, a part that might continue to use its influence
causing you to continue to smoke.

If that should happen, if you should experience any
desire whatever to smoke, it simply means this work
is not complete, not that this work is a failure. Should
that happen, we will interact with Centrum again during our next session to identify and resolve whatever
form that influence might take.

This negative
response was
not expected. An
affirmative response
is the norm this
early in treatment,
requiring each
remaining identified
part to be educated/
persuaded to change
its influence.

Note that in normal
conversation, the
question would have
provoked an elaborate
answer. Here, Pat has
spontaneously slipped
into trance and the
characteristic of
energy conservation
is demonstrated.

Yet, it is possible to conduct a test here and now, by using your imagination. Pat, as we have been working you have spontaneously slipped into a trance state. Please take advantage of that state, and the imaginative ability it provides, to project yourself into a series of situations in which, in the past, you would have wanted to smoke. Do that and see if you experience any desire whatsoever to smoke while in those situations. *There was no desire. I did it three times.*

THIRD SESSION – one week later

How did it go for you during the past week? *I am still smoking, but a lot less often than before, and with a lot less desire. I am down to one or two a day. And, I've been practicing self-hypnosis twice a day also.*

Very good. Now let's get back to work. Centrum, are you aware that you have continued to smoke? YES Centrum, are you willing to continue this work, with the objective of completely eliminating all desire to smoke? YES Centrum, please re-investigate, set the stage as you did last time, and let me know when you have completed the task. COMPLETE

Centrum, please identify the remaining part, or parts, that have continued to influence you to smoke. COMPLETE Centrum, did you identify one or more such parts? YES How many such parts did you identify? ONE

Centrum, please repeat the protocol you used last week. First, listen. Then educate that part about your present life situation. Let that part understand the negative consequences of its influence. "Grow that part up," Centrum, and let me know when you have done so by the word "complete." COMPLETE Centrum, were you successful in that task? YES, STRESS

Pat might have reported an increase in smoking frequency. In either case there has been behavioral change, a strong indication that the therapy is having an effect.

Note the increased efficiency with which Centrum works. The details of steps have been learned, and you need only request the task and step out of the way. If there are other goals to be accomplished, Centrum will be able to do the work in far briefer time.

Centrum, please provide conscious understanding of the work you just did, doing so by memories, the chalkboard, or by whatever means is appropriate, and let me know when you have completed the task. COMPLETE Pat, are you now satisfied that you are in fact an ex-smoker? *Yes*

Centrum, I again ask that you search the unconscious domain of your mind, to identify any part of your mind, that for any reason whatsoever, might cause you to continue to smoke. Let me know when you have completed that task. COMPLETE Centrum, did you identify any remaining part or parts of your mind? NO Centrum, are you now an ex-smoker? YES

A follow-up at three-months revealed that Pat had not smoked since the last session and had no desire to do so.

Barbara – A Case of Anxiety and Libido – In-Class Demonstration

Barbara volunteered as a demonstration subject in my hypnosis class at the University of California, San Diego (UCSD) School of Medicine. The following transcription is of a DVD that was recorded at the time and copies of which are available via my website. Barbara had read my introduction booklet (Yager, 1985) prior to the demonstration, which lasted about two hours, and the course of treatment went unusually smoothly. This transcription also includes interactions with class members, which are noted in a sans serif typeface.

Class, this young lady's name is Barbara. Barbara has volunteered to be here and she has volunteered to be recorded. She has a problem that she'd like fixed and I hope that's what she gets out of this, and I hope you get more than that. So, tell me a little bit about you, Barbara. *A little bit about me? Or my problems?*

How old are you Barbara? *I'm 33.*

Thirty-three, is that old? *I'm starting to feel old.* (laughs) *I'm getting wrinkles right here.* (points to face)

No, no, no, no, no. *I'm 33 years old, I'm a single mother. I have three children.*

Three children? *10, 7, and 5.*

Wow! *Yeah. Two boys and a girl. I'm a massage therapist. It's what I do for a living for now. I want to get into acupuncture, that's where I'm headed.*

I've supervised a Marriage and Family Therapist applicant by the name of Bill Muller. Ever hear of Muller College of Massage? *Yes.*

He established that college. *Oh, okay!*

I supervised him as he was seeking licensure. It was an amazing thing to share a wall with him, with a thin wall between us when he did massage therapy. I was just astounded at the degree to which emotion can be elicited by massage. I had no idea that was possible. So he really educated me, too. What else might I need to know about you? What kind of person are you? *I can be very outgoing, and I can also close up around people. I'm a very driven person, but I always come up against walls that keep me from doing what I want to do, and I feel … defeated a lot.*

Do you know what those walls are? *A lot of it has to do with, I think, how I feel about myself. I have a lot of self-beliefs that I want to change to be able to succeed in business, family and relationships. It's all mental, I just don't know how to change it.*

Well, I hope to teach you the most effective way I know to change it. See, this is an interesting therapy approach because of several factors, but one of the factors is that I will not really be very involved in the content of what you're dealing with. I'm on the out-

Rapport comes from learning about and sensitizing yourself to the other person. You know when you are there when you find yourself 'feeling like' you understand the other person, and vice versa.

side. I'm just a guide for this process, you have to do all the work. It all happens over there. I just sit back and coast. And, at the same time I'm guiding you to use this technique, you're learning how to use it. Now, we don't make very good self therapists … I don't think we can be objective about ourselves. But, there's a lot of things we can do. So, if you can do it, go for it! Nothing can be lost. So you'll be learning a new skill here, okay? *Okay.*

Okay, now … please tell me about the problem. *I deal with a lot of anxiety. Generally speaking, out of one to ten it's usually a five, and I feel it in my stomach area, I feel it in my gut, I feel it in my chest, I have breathing problems, it's hard to breathe deeply. When I get into a relationship it gets much worse, so I lose weight and I'm not healthy, so I have to get out of the relationship so I can get healthy and gain weight again. I've had a history of abusive relationships and I'm assuming that's probably part of it.*

As a child, you mean? *Yeah, like my relationships with my dad … he was scary, I think that's where a lot of my self-esteem issues come from, not feeling lovable or worthy or deserving. I carry that with me. And then, as I got older, intimate relationships were often with people who were verbally or emotionally abusive. So, I need a new picker, so I can pick 'em better. (Laughs) I wake up in the morning, I go throughout my day, doing the dishes or whatever, and I notice I'm like this (clenches fists) and my mind is constantly going, and I'm feeling like I'm not doing enough, or not … good enough, or constantly, you know it's this constant … depression and anxiety go hand in hand with me. My mom says, "Go take a walk and enjoy your day outside," and it's like I go take a walk but I'm not enjoying anything because I feel I've missed the boat, I feel like I can't engage in life, and be a part of it, and just relax and enjoy day-to-day life. There's something that's unresolved, I feel like something needs to be resolved and I don't know what that is. And I just want to be able to enjoy my children, I just want to enjoy everyday life and I feel like I've*

Barbara is very intelligent and articulate. It's easy to understand where she comes from on issues and the meaning of her expressions. This characteristic has high value in ST.

The goals she is presenting are still very generalized; they must be clarified and simplified.

*missed the boat. Life is happening and I can't engage … it.
And it's very frustrating.*

Okay, have you ever, as far as you can remember,
enjoyed the kind of constructive relationship you
really want? *Um, no. I mean, I'm really close with my
mom. I enjoy my relationship with her. Intimate relationships, no. There's just that constant … you know, I have it
right now … there's just this constant tight feeling and I
just go from one thing to the next and I'm just waiting to
die. Like I'm just going from one thing to the next thing, to
the next thing, until life is over and I want to slow down
and enjoy what I'm doing, I want to enjoy the process of
learning and I want to be able to do that, and I haven't
been able to do that.*

You're entitled. *Yeah, so the other issue with intimate
relationships … Sex is a big issue for me, um … I don't
enjoy it, I'm not comfortable, I can't relax, I'm nervous the
whole time, and it really sucks.*

So it goes over into the sexual domain, too? *Yeah,
and I think … I have a vague memory from when I was
really little, I got out of the apartment and I was knocking
on people's doors, and I think I was like 3, and some guy
invited me in, and I remember … he wanted me to rub
lotion on his legs, and then I go blank. I don't remember
anything else after that. And I've had some instances of
molestation as a teenager too, so I don't know if that probably has something to do with it, the fear factor.*

We'll find out. *I want to resolve that issue as well.*

You speak of being anxious right now … you know
the zero to ten scale? Where are you right now? *It hard
because I'm used to it, but, well, because my stomach hurts
and everything … probably like a four?*

Do you know anything about hypnosis? *I don't, really,
I mean, I think that most of things people say about it
probably aren't true, so … I know that much.*

That's very probable, yes. The master–slave relation-ship is not true. I ask that question because as I guide you to do these things, I think you'll probably spon-taneously slip into trance, the trance state of hypnosis. We all do this; what we call hypnosis is a natural experience. And that's probably going to happen. Now, sometimes people are a little … put off by the idea, they don't want to lose control, or something like that. *If it helps me relax, I think I'll be all for it!* (laughs)

Well, it's a way of gaining control, and I think you'll find that to be true. Now, I think it's a valuable skill to have to be able to go into trance ourselves. So I want to teach you self-hypnosis. Just take the time to do that. It's very easy. Truly, there's nothing to going into trance. Nevertheless, to get there yourself on a premeditated basis, it helps to have a little protocol to go through; a few steps to take. I want to guide you to take four simple little steps. And anytime you want the experience again, just repeat those four simple lit-tle steps. Okay? *Okay.*

Any concerns you have about going into trance? *Just that my brain will try to fight it.*

Your brain will try to fight it? *I feel like I won't be able to do it.*

Well, okay. *I guess I'll just try and let it happen.*

That's the whole key. Going into trance is kind of like relaxing. If I ask you to relax, what am I asking you to do? I'm not really asking you to do anything. And that's true about going into trance. You set the stage for what I'll guide you to do, but once there, you just let it happen. Okay? Now, the four steps I want you to take, I want to go over in advance. Step 1 – I will ask that you close your eyes in just a moment. Step 2 – I will ask that you use your imagination, and play a little game with yourself, and I'll guide you to do these steps, don't worry about all that. The game

I teach all of my patients self-hypnosis, usually before using ST.

This is the procedure I use unless there is reason not to. This simple, four-step protocol is the most effective for most people.

These are the words I typically use. Different words that convey the same meaning may be more appropriate for you.

is to pretend those eyes won't open. Step 3 – while you're pretending those eyes won't open, I will invite you to try to open them. What you'll find is, as long as you pretend they won't, they won't open. This is a very unusual experience for almost everybody. And, I explain it as a simple little physical demonstration of the authority of our imagination, which I've come to believe is the most powerful, single influence on the way we experience life. And, even as you're doing this, you will know – there won't be any question in your mind – that you can stop anytime and open your eyes if you want to. And if you need to do that, I want you to do that. I want you to know that YOU are in control, and for many reasons. I don't want control. Okay? And if you do that, then I'll just take you back to Step 1, because I want you to have that skill. Sound like a good approach? *(nods head)*

Go ahead and take Step 1. Close your eyes. And now, take Step 2 – make believe, pretend those eyes – well, maybe pretend you're a little girl again, and you're playing a game, and part of the game is that you have eyes that won't open. It's like they're glued closed. Pretend those eyes are glued closed, and simply will not open at all. And now, while pretending they won't open, I invite you to try to open them. Physically, I want to see you exercise your eye muscles. Ahh, very good. Now, this is the fourth step – relax your eyes, and relax your whole body with that, simply permit this experience to be yours. You see, Barbara, I assure you, what you are experiencing, right now, at this moment, this is what we call the trance state of hypnosis. I presume you're experiencing this at a fairly light level. What I do know is that as you experience this state, with the passage of time, you'll go into the state more deeply. As the moments go by, you'll become more and more relaxed into this state, more and more completely relaxed. Now, the first thing I want you to be aware of, Barbara, is that you are aware. You hear my voice, you are aware of yourself, anything you choose to be aware of. And that will always be true, no matter how deeply you ever go into this state. You will be aware. And to the extent you are aware, you are in control. Now, there are some changes that take place as we go into trance. Muscles all through your body are permitted to relax, your body becomes quiet and still, and to some extent, your mind becomes quiet and still. You don't stop thinking, you can think about whatever you want to think about. At the same time, however, you're probably not thinking about problems or inclined to worry about anything. And, another very valuable change that happens is that, while in trance, we are able to divorce ourselves from negative emotions. We use the term 'disassociate' from emotions. You can remember, if you choose to, you can remember what it felt like to be anxious, and angry, but right now, right now, you're not. And that has some very powerful, positive benefits, both physically and mentally. Mentally, largely because you're able to think clearly without the emotional bias. Now as we work together using the technique you read about in the little book, I think you'll probably spontaneously slip into this state. And that's fine, that's good, I just wanted you to know what was happening. And, when you practice this on your own, which I encourage you to do, you can go into the state as often as you wish. You can go into the state for as long as you wish. And all you need to do is repeat those four, simple little steps, and you'll go right back into trance. You'll close your eyes, you pretend they won't open, you test them to be sure they won't open, as you did, and finally, you relax them. Everything that just happened you did, I'm just a guide, I taught you how, and you don't need me anymore. This is a skill that you can pursue on your own as you wish. And when you rouse from trance, you bring back to the normal waking state the benefits; the good parts of being in trance. That can last for a long time. And if need be, of course you can go back into trance and reinforce it. So, in a moment, when I ask you to rouse yourself from trance I want you to bring back all of the positive things you can identify about it now. And, if you will please, at your own pace, Barbara, at your own pace, if you will please rouse yourself from trance, open your eyes, and notice how good you feel. *Wow!*

Like that? *(Nods, breathing deeply)*

...

And, where are you on the zero to ten scale right now? *Like a one. A one or a two.*

Okay, now, I want to shift gears. I want to talk about the technique you read about in my little book. And having briefly reviewed that to set the stage, I'm going to jump right into it. Now, to do this best, I'm going to ask that you give me an expression. A simple, concise, complete goal. What do you want to accomplish here today? *I guess I want to relearn …*

Would you like an example or two? *I want to get rid of my anxiety, I know that.*

Alright, okay, primary goal – get rid of your anxiety. *Yeah, the general anxiety.*

As a secondary goal to that, might it be accurate to say that … I don't mean to suggest this, I mean it as a kind of an example I want from you – that you be free to what? *Engage in a healthy relationship? Intimately?*

So, free yourself from any barriers to doing this. *Yes.*

Anything else? *To be able to have sex and enjoy it? (laughs)*

Okay, great! That's a good one, it's a powerful one. Okay, now … as you read in the little book … this technique I propose to guide you to use is based on certain assumptions. The basic assumption is that we are conditioned by life experiences to be as we are. Do you have any problem with that concept? *No, I*

Since anxiety is expressed as the most important goal, it will be addressed first.

These will be the next two goals addressed.

This marks the beginning of the actual treatment.

understand. I don't have a problem with that. Well, I have a problem with how I was conditioned.

That's what we have to find out, you see. Now, I don't think there are any limits to that conditioning business. I think anyone could have been conditioned to be anything. But that's my biased opinion. But I am very clear in my professional opinion that your problems we've been speaking of are not genetic; they are a consequence of life experience. We are conditioned during those experiences to experience life as we do today. And our basic task here is reconditioning. Let me give you an illustration, an example. If we terrify a little kid in a dark place, it's very logical that she would associate fear with the dark, and then be afraid when you turn the lights out. If a dog bites a child, it's reasonable that the child would learn to be afraid of dogs. It only becomes a problem if it becomes extended over time. That would be called a phobia in diagnosing an adult. Well, I think your anxiety – I'm going to focus on them one at a time, I can't promise to get through them all, but we're going to address one at a time, and go as far as we can, and then, as I promised, I will follow up with you privately. The other assumption is that we have mental capacities that, in all probability, we don't know we have. Some people seem to have a sense that they have a higher level of consciousness, a 'super-consciousness' or something, but most people don't ever think about that kind of thing. But I think you have those abilities. And I propose to guide you to resolve these abilities to solve those problems. I refer to this higher level ability as Centrum. For convenience. *I read that.*

> Making this statement seems to bring reality to the concept of conditioning.

And so when I address a question to Centrum, I'm not addressing you consciously, I'm addressing Centrum, at a super-conscious level. It seems that every time we learn something new, be it a skill, or to be afraid of something, or a behavior, whatever it may be, something is there now that wasn't there before. Something was added. Whatever that something is

> Again, the typical words I use that you may choose to replace.

(that I can't adequately define), except that it has to be there, I refer to as a 'part'. I think the unconscious/subconscious domain of our minds is largely made up of the collection of these lessons and influences, these parts that we have accumulated during life. Now, fortunately, a majority of these parts are good stuff. But every once in awhile, we learn something … negative. We learn to feel anxious, for example. I think there's a part in your mind that causes you to feel anxious, because it feels anxious. Our task, then, is to identify that part, and re-educate that part. I think that part is stuck back in time; it knows only what you knew when that part came into existence. It hasn't kept up like the rest of your mind has. Our task is to bring that part up to speed, to inform, to educate it. And while we can do that one part at a time, we can do that far more efficiently – more accurately spoken – YOU can do it far more efficiently by relying on Centrum's ability. Assuming Centrum is willing to do this – very high odds – Centrum can do it while we're thinking what question to ask. So, you have any questions now? You've read the book, you've heard me narrate about it. *I have no questions.*

Do you have the key so far? *Yes.*

Now, I mentioned my role in all of this is be a guide, and to be a guide, I have to be able to communicate with your Centrum. Your Centrum can hear me now. What's missing is the communication in the other direction; I need to know what Centrum says. I can't hear your Centrum. And that's where your conscious role comes into play. That's where the chalkboard comes into play. That's the preferred way. Not the only way, but the preferred way, for a number of reasons. So it becomes your job, in other words, to consciously create an image of a chalkboard, and then communicate to me what Centrum writes on the chalkboard, as opposed to what you might consciously think should be written there. *That's where I'm afraid I might get tripped up. What if I'm making it up?*

Here I begin setting up communications with Centrum and I begin to stress the essential importance of her communicating, literally, the words on the chalkboard.

71

Most of the answers will be obvious. Most of what Centrum says, you will know to be true and accurate. But, some of the answers may not make sense. You won't understand them, and you just may out and out disagree with some of those answers. And Barbara, that's all okay, as long as you will tell me what the answers are, as opposed to what you might think the answers should be. The moment you fill in a blank, or change an answer, we start spinning wheels. Alright? *Okay.*

Now, this requires some mental discipline on your part. *So, whatever appears on the chalkboard …*

That's what I want to hear from you. The guiding rule is this: Anytime I preface a question with name Centrum, the next words I hope to hear from you are what's on the chalkboard. Do you think you can do that? As long as you do that, we'll go charging down the right path. Now, set up your chalkboard, if you will. *Okay, do I close my eyes?*

Most people do, but not everybody. Okay, close your eyes and create the image of a chalkboard and let me know when you have it. *I have it.*

I ask that Centrum, your Centrum, indicate willingness to communicate with me by these means. Please indicate that, Centrum, by writing the word "yes", Y-E-S. Right on the chalkboard. Let me know when it's there. *Okay, it's there.*

You might, as you pointed out very reasonably, you might say "it says 'yes'. But I can easily imagine a chalkboard that says 'yes', or 'no', or whatever you want. How do I know that it's Centrum?" Part of the answer is that if, in fact, you put it there, you can take it away. However, if Centrum wrote that word "yes", in all probability you will not be able to erase it. Is it still there? *Yes.*

Now, I invite you to try and erase it. Still there? *Mm-hm.*

Okay. Now I want to give you another little exercise to further demonstrate that something different is going on here. Centrum, please erase the word "yes", and replace it with a different word. This time, Centrum, I ask you to select a word that will surprise you consciously. Maybe some off-the-wall word. CHERRY

Are you satisfied that you did not consciously come up with that word and put it there? *Mm-hm.*

Okay, the only purpose for that little exercise is to give you first-person awareness that something is going on here. Okay now, Centrum – are you aware of your conscious concern about this anxiety? How it's interfering with your life? Are you, Centrum, aware that that's happening? YES

This is the opening question; the beginning of treatment.

Centrum, are you willing to cooperate here, to do some work as I guide you and teach you how, with the objective of eliminating that anxiety from your life? It's unfortunate, it's dysfunctional and should be eliminated. Are you willing to cooperate in eliminating that anxiety, Centrum? YES

Engaging Centrum in the work by asking if it is willing to work.

Centrum, I need to ask a couple of questions just so I can know that we are on common ground. Centrum, do you have the ability to access memories of events that have taken place in your life? YES

And do you also have the ability to communicate with other parts of your mind? YES

A "no" answer would have required that I interrupt the ideal sequence of events to guide Centrum to awareness that the ability is actually present.

Okay. Well, Centrum, I believe you have abilities I don't even know how to begin to talk about. These abilities you have, I ask you to use them now. Specifically, I ask that you conduct an investigation, there in the unconscious domain. An investigation into the roots of the anxiety. Looking for those experiences when you learned to feel anxious. In other words, Centrum, identify those parts of your mind that are causing you to feel anxious. Is that request clear to you, Centrum? YES

"Is it clear to you?" is an exceedingly important question! "Wheel spinning" can result without it.

Then, Centrum, please do that now; conduct that investigation, doing so, Centrum, with or without conscious awareness as you deem appropriate. And let me know by writing the word "complete" on the chalkboard when you have completed that task. COMPLETE

"With or without conscious awareness" makes it possible for Centrum to protect the patient, even while doing the necessary work.

Centrum, do you believe you now understand how, why, where and when you learned to feel anxious? YES

Centrum, is there any reason you should not have this information consciously? NO

Unconscious objection is not uncommon.

Okay, and Centrum – I will be guiding you, assuming you're willing to cooperate, I will be guiding you to identify those parts that came into existence back then. Those parts that are still anxious, causing you to feel anxious. First to identify them, and then to do some reconditioning of those parts. The first task I ask of you, then, is that you identify those parts, in preparation for communicating with them, that you identify those parts of your mind that are causing you to feel anxious these days. And to let me know by the word "complete" that you have done so. Centrum, was my request clear? COMPLETE

Okay. Centrum, did you identify one or more parts of your mind that are anxious, and causing you to feel anxious? YES

Centrum, how many parts did you identify? FIVE

Okay. Centrum, I presume that means there were five particular experiences that you had in life, in consequence of which, you learned to feel anxious. Now,

Centrum – I ask that you select one of those parts, perhaps the first that came into existence. Select one of those parts, and communicate with the part in this way. I neglected to ask a question, Centrum. Are you in communication with all five of those parts? YES

Okay, then select one of those parts, and communicate with that part in this way. First, Centrum, I ask that you listen to the part. Find out from the part what it believes, and why it believes what it believes. Learn why the part is influencing you to continue to be anxious. And then, Centrum, based on that information, I ask that you educate the part about present reality. You see, Centrum, that part is stuck back there in time. It is functioning on the basis of what it knew when it came into existence. It's unaware of present life, and the effects of its influence. I'm asking, Centrum, that you educate the part about all of that. Persuade the part to support your life needs now. Is that request clear to you, Centrum? YES

Then please, Centrum, persuade that part to your way of thinking, and let me know when you have done so by writing the word "complete". COMPLETE

Okay. Centrum, were you successful in that task? YES

Okay. Then Centrum, I ask that you select a second part and repeat the same protocol. First, listen, and then educate. Centrum, what you're doing here is reconditioning. So recondition that second part, and let me know when you have finished that task. COMPLETE

Centrum, were you successful with that second part? YES

Then Centrum, I ask that you repeat that same protocol with each of the three remaining parts that you have identified. One at a time, Centrum. Work with one at a time. Listen, learn what you need to know, then educate. Then, when you have completed the task with one part, repeat the protocol with the next and then the next. And then let me know when you have completed communicating with those three parts of your mind. COMPLETE

Centrum, were you successful with all three of those parts? YES

Now, Centrum, it is so commonly true that when one issue has been resolved, it is then, and only then, possible to identify some other issues that need to be addressed. Centrum, I ask that you search to identify any remaining parts of your mind, part or parts of your mind, that have in the past, or might in the future, cause you to feel anxious. Centrum, please conduct that search, and let me know when you have completed the task. COMPLETE

And, Centrum, did you identify one or more additional parts? YES

How many did you identify? FOUR

Then Centrum, I ask that you repeat that same protocol with each of those four parts. Again, one at a time. Recondition each, persuade each to support present life needs, and let me know when you have completed that task. COMPLETE

Centrum, were you successful in reconditioning all four of those parts? YES

Then Centrum, please search once again. Perhaps there is still some other part of your mind that feels anxious for some reason, and might influence you to feel the anxiety consciously. Search yet again, Centrum. Identify any remaining parts, and let me know when you have done so. COMPLETE

Guide Centrum to search for remaining parts, and resolve them as they are uncovered, until there are no more. Always, always do this ...

And Centrum, were you successful with all of those parts? YES

Then Centrum, search again. Perhaps there is still some part of your mind. Let me know when you've completed the search. COMPLETE

Did you identify *any* remaining part? NO

Okay. Great work, Centrum. Thank you. And now, Centrum, I say to you that I do not know whether you have had, or have not had, conscious awareness of the work that you, Centrum, have been doing. So I need to know at this point, Centrum. Do you now have full conscious memory, understanding, of the work that you have been doing? NO

Okay, Centrum, in my opinion, there is real value in having this understanding consciously. In having the memories of those nine events, or whatever it was, so that you can consciously comprehend the process whereby you learned to feel anxious. Like the kid learning to feel fear about dogs. Same philosophy; same kind of reasoning. On the other hand, Centrum, there may be some reason that you should not know this consciously. Some part of your mind might believe that this would not be good. So what I ask, Centrum, do you, you Centrum, believe that it is in your best interest that you have all of this information consciously? YES

Centrum, does any part of your mind disagree? YES

And Centrum, are you in communication with that part? YES

Then Centrum, communicate with that part again. Listen, find out what that part believes and why. Centrum, you might even change your mind. Listen to the part, Centrum. Find out what that part's objection is. Find out what it's all about, and let me know when you know by the word "complete". COMPLETE

Centrum, do you still think it's in your best interest to have this knowledge consciously? NO.

Note that this is a change in Centrum's opinion. Centrum too is capable of learning and changing.

Okay, well then tell me, Barbara. I'm addressing you by your first name, I'm speaking to you consciously, I want your conscious opinion about this, not a response from Centrum. What do you think about that consciously, Barbara? *I want to know.*

You want to know? It's important to you to know? *Yes.*

Okay. Centrum, there is a strong conscious desire to know. Would it be okay, Centrum, for you to be consciously aware of some collection of satisfying aspects of this, to satisfy that conscious desire? Would that much be okay? YES

And, Centrum, does any part object to that? NO

Then Centrum, please elevate that understanding, that knowledge, those memories, whatever's involved, to consciousness now. And let me know, Centrum, by the word "complete", that you have elevated all of the information that's appropriate at this time. COMPLETE

Now back to you consciously, Barbara. Did you get some knowledge this time? Did you learn some things about you? *No.*

Well, okay. Centrum, no knowledge got though. Centrum, is some part of your mind blocking any of this information from being made conscious? YES

Centrum, are you in communication with that part? YES

Barbara wants to know, Centrum has agreed to provide the information, and yet none came through. There can be only one explanation: Some part is resisting conscious awareness for some reason.

78

Then Centrum, please communicate with that part. That part, too, Centrum, is well-intended. It's probably protecting you, taking the position that it wouldn't be good to go through all of that again, or something of that nature. Well, I submit that you survived the original experience. You can certainly survive the memory of that experience now, especially with the additional coping abilities and such that you have now. So I ask, Centrum, that you do all you know to permit the memories to become conscious. And let me know, by the word "complete", that you have done so. COMPLETE

Centrum, were you successful in persuading that part to permit the memories? YES

Then Centrum, once again I ask that you elevate those memories and information to consciousness, doing so now. And let me know when you have done so. COMPLETE

Were you successful in getting those memories across this time, Centrum? YES

And, back to you consciously now, Barbara. Are you satisfied with that? Does that knowledge satisfy your need to know, or do you want more? *I'm confused.*

Okay, Centrum. *Am I supposed to be remembering stuff? Like is stuff supposed to popping into my conscious mind about …*

Remember that Centrum agreed to reveal only "a collection of satisfying aspects" of the original experience. Barbara seems to have expected more.

That typically happens, did that happen to you? Even though it was confusing, did information happen? Did you get a memory, for example … *Yeah.*

Tell me that memory, and I'll give you a possible explanation about it. *I just remember when I was … I think I was around 8 or 9, I was at an after-school program and they had a rabbit that I would go in and feed, and pet, and stuff like that, and that's what popped into my head. This is where I … I just don't know …*

Well, I want to point out – that memory is now being considered from the perspective of knowledge that you have now, as a young adult. You see, Barbara, things have an effect on us, no question about that, events have an effect on us. And that effect is dependent on where we are in life, what we know, what coping skills we have, and on and on. When you were that age, you didn't have near the coping skills you have today as an adult. So, in all probability, it's okay to remember that memory, and the consequence of whatever happened, here and now, under these safe conditions. It will not be experienced negatively. It won't have the same effect on you. Am I making logical sense to you? Centrum, am I making logical sense to you? YES

This level of difficulty is unusual.

Then Centrum, please communicate that to that part that is resisting the memories. See if you can persuade that part to permit the entire memory, all of the information, and let me know when you have done what you know to do. COMPLETE

Okay. Centrum, were you successful in persuading the part to permit the full knowledge? YES

Good. Then Centrum, let the information be complete consciously. COMPLETE

Okay. Barbara, are you now satisfied? Does it all come together for you now? Or is there still more you would like to know? *Am I supposed to be consciously aware of all of those things that …*

All of this effort to achieve conscious awareness of the cause may not be necessary. It was pursued only to satisfy her expressed, conscious desire to know.

You may be aware of all of it in a more general sense or you may be aware of each of those specific things that Centrum has asked. *'Cause um, I would see a number on the chalkboard and I wouldn't be consciously aware of what exactly those things were, I'm just relaying to you what things I'm seeing on the chalkboard.*

What I'm talking about here is a cause–effect phenomenon. In a given situation as a child, when you had some experience, you understood that experience from the perspective of the knowledge you had as that child. You learned to be afraid of the dark, for example. Well, that doesn't make sense to the adult line of reasoning, but it made very good sense back then. I think you'll find the same thing true here. For example, can you tell me what the first event was, that taught you to be anxious? Can you tell me about that experience? Do you know what that was? *I don't know what it is, but what keeps popping into my head is my dad.*

Your dad? *Mm-hm.*

Okay. I have an idea that Centrum is being a little cautious, and not giving you wholesale information, and I am back to your conscious opinion now – would you want to know whatever it is having to do with your dad? *Yes.*

Maybe he did something stupid. Would you consciously want to know? *Yes.*

Centrum, are you willing to oblige? YES

Then Centrum, please do so. Now, it is not necessary that you express what comes to your mind. Just be aware that what happened, and aware of the effect it had on you then, and aware of the ongoing influence, which is probably the anxiety. Let me know when you have that completed the task by the word "complete". COMPLETE

Centrum, please provide conscious awareness of the remaining nine items. Or eight items, I mean. OKAY, COMPLETE

And are you now consciously satisfied with all of that? Did you get the picture better now? You understand how, why, where, and when you learned to be anxious? *Yes.*

Do any of those influences still have a role in your life, a positive role in your life? Do they serve any purpose in your life today as an adult? *No.*

Centrum, do you agree with that answer? YES

Then Centrum, please communicate that concept to every part of your mind, so that there can be universal support going on in there. COMPLETE

Okay, very good. Now Barbara, I want you to be aware that you have spontaneously slipped into trance as we have been working. Do you recognize it? *Yes.*

Okay. I want to ask now that you rouse yourself, and let's discuss this a little bit. *Hi.*

Hi. What do you think? Are you through with that one? *Yeah, I um ... it's interesting ... I'm not quite sure how it works, I'm sure there's a lot of stuff going on that I'm not consciously aware of it, which is fine for me.*

Note that she did not have conscious awareness of all material addressed by Centrum.

Okay. Is there any aspect of what you just learned that you want to talk about? Whether it has to do with the process or content of what you just learned? Or anything else, any aspect at all you want to talk about? *I guess just when I felt pressured, like I felt when ... I felt like I had to recall something, I wasn't sure if I was recalling the right thing or if it was coming up; if I needed to recall it. It made me nervous, I felt nervous about that.*

I did not wish to impose a requirement on her to reveal private information in the presence of the class.

Well, I'm not asking you to do this, I'm asking you, would it be possible if you wanted to, could you articulate, could you describe, to lay out a story, this is how I came to be anxious ... Would that be possible? *Yeah.*

I'm not asking you to do that, don't misunderstand me. *Yes. Do you want me to? Are you asking me to do it?*

I'm going to deviate here. I'm going to talk to the class for a moment …

I want you in the class to hear loud and clear that she was successful in resolving her problem as I guided her to do the work. The work is complete and I do not know what the cause of her problem was. I was not involved in content and that is in direct contradiction with what therapists are taught about doing psycho-therapy. We're supposed to be involved in the content, evaluating and arriving at conclusions. Now, it would be nice if there were some way to test whether or not the problem is actually resolved, if the work is actually complete. Of course, the final test is in the real world, yet it would be of value to test completeness – at least provisionally – now. And, there may be such a test.

The next step we're going to take here is this, I'm going to ask you to use your imagination. Slip into trance, maybe … at least close your eyes, and really get into the imaginary process. Imagine yourself in some situation in which in the past you would have really felt anxious. And tell me what happens. *I'm having a really hard time with confrontation, and so I'm imagining myself confronting somebody, and I could see myself doing it without getting too anxious.*

Well, that's a pretty positive indicator. And for the class I say, had there been any reservation about that success, it would have indicated that the work was still not complete, there's still some part of her mind that's still involved, and still might cause the anxiety to continue. But, this is what we have to go by at this given point in time. Given her life exposure out there, and then she'll be able to tell us whether the work is complete or not.

And I say to you, Barbara, that if you should find some situation in which you are still anxious, it doesn't mean this work wasn't successful, it just means that the work is not complete. I want to hear from you, I want to find that hidden part and resolve it also. Now, would you be willing to answer questions from the class? You don't have to answer, but any answers you would be willing to give them ... would you be willing to respond? *Yes, sure.*

Okay, guys. What are your questions? No questions?

(Student A) I have a question. How was your experience imagining your childhood? *That was easy for me ... um, what was hard at first was I didn't know if I was consciously putting "yes" on the chalkboard, but I just got used to it. I guess just being in a relaxed state, I could just see it appear, and I was able to separate my conscious mind from it and it was just an automatic thing that was happening. But for me, I'm a very visual person, so it was easy for me to visualize the chalkboard.*

(Student A) Were you pretty satisfied that it was an unconscious communication, or ... *At first, no. Because like I said, I though maybe my brain ... my consciousness was getting in the way. But after a couple of times, I was satisfied that it was my subconscious ... that it was a subconscious phenomena that was occurring. It's kind of hard to explain ... like sometimes I wouldn't even ... like one time a "no" came into my head, and I didn't agree with it, and I was like, "what?", and then you (Dr. Yager) asked me consciously and I didn't agree with it, but it was there written on the chalkboard. It was interesting. How dare my own mind tell me no? Yeah, it was weird ... I wanted it to say yes. But it didn't.*

(Student B) Was there any point during the process that you felt your anxiety increasing? *Yeah, when I was asked to recall memories. Like when he was asking Centrum to let things surface. And nothing was really surfacing, so it was kind of a panic thing, like I was supposed to be remembering something and I'm not, so that was kind of like a performance anxiety thing, I guess. I didn't know what say, or I didn't know if I was doing it right, or was something supposed to be coming up. So that was the part that made me feel anxious, when I had to consciously answer about retrieving memoires, I guess. Yeah.*

(Student C) How did that resolve? So you felt anxious at that moment, then what happened? *Um, he (Dr. Yager) asked me … I think … 'cause something did pop into my head but I didn't make sense of why that would pop into my head. Um, so … him asking me what it was, and then it was that memory of me when I was feeding that rabbit or whatever. But, through the whole thing, I got a more … a clearer picture, more of the story of why I have this anxiety. And a lot of it was memories that I already remember. Like I remember a lot of my childhood, and why I would be anxious when that happened … I can't remember any like … I do remember specific things, but it kind of integrated it, I guess? You know, you have it put into all of these fragmented pieces and just kind of integrating them together into a story of why. So when I was able to say "yes, I understand" why I was anxious – not just specific instances – but why. I have a picture in my mind of why, and that was easier to talk about, I guess.*

(Student D) Were there any surprises? *Um, yeah I was surprised that I could see things on the chalkboard and know that it wasn't really my conscious mind doing it, that surprised me 'cause I thought I would fight it, and just be writing things on the chalkboard; my conscious mind writing things on there.*

(Student D) Did any memories come up that you hadn't remembered before? *No.*

(Student E) Your fear of confrontation … do you feel like that's resolved? *When I was imagining confronting somebody?*

(Student E) For instance, before that exercise that you had to imagine an instance where you were in a confrontation, and you dealt with it in a way that made you anxious ... because you said that confrontations make you kind of anxious. Had that happened to you before, where you thought of that scenario? *It would always make me anxious. Thinking about confronting, yeah. So that was cool. So now I'm kind of like ... wanting to confront somebody to see if it's real.*

(Student F) There seemed to be some hesitation when you imagined confrontation, or ... there seemed to be hesitation, because I was trying to read or interpret your body language. Was there a bit of ...? *No, I was just trying to figure it out as quickly as I could; to think of a scenario where I would feel anxious, and I was just kind of flipping through my mind to think of what would have ... and then I thought, "confrontation", and then I just kind of imagined ... you know, I have a particular issue with somebody, going over to their house, and confronting them on it, and normally doing that would cause me great anxiety and I would just avoid this person. But I was able to imagine doing it, so ...*

(Student G) In particular, was there pretty much no, or little anxiety? *Yeah, there was little anxiety in just telling a person how I felt, and not feeling bad or guilty for how I felt.*

At which point was this? *When you asked me to imagine ...*

There at the end? *Yeah.*

There was anxiety? *No, there wasn't. He was asking me if there was, and there wasn't.*

Oh, oh. Okay.

(Student H) Do you feel like you could actually go over to their house? *Yeah, I could talk to them and just tell them how I feel and to feel like I'm okay for owning those feelings and not bad, or I shouldn't feel guilty, or that how they feel is my responsibility, or that I don't have a right to feel that way, and I can be okay with that and it's okay if they don't understand. The anxiety is just not there. It's kind of interesting; weird.*

(Student H) Did you say it was weird? *Yeah, it's just interesting.*

(Student H) Why is it weird? *'Cause normally I'm so wrapped up and worried about what the outcome's going to be that it just makes me so anxious, so it's weird to me to think of something like that and not really worry about what the outcome's going to be.*

(Student H) I don't know if this is you, or if this is just the decrease in anxiety overall, but I noticed that you are speaking differently than you were when you first came in. *Now that you mention it, yeah. I'm more calm, calmer.*

Aware that you're thinking differently now.

(Student I) Were you aware of all of those nine items? *Not at all, and that's kind of why, or what made me feel anxious 'cause I didn't know if I was supposed to be recalling exactly what those things were, or when he asked Centrum … I was thinking "two", but when he actually asked the question, "five" appeared on the chalkboard, so I'm like five, 'cause that's what it said … I didn't know what those five items were specifically. I can tell you five things that I know probably made me anxious when I was a child, but I don't know if that was what it was …*

(Student I) You don't know if those were the five Centrum actually dealt with? *Exactly, yeah. I don't know specifically, I mean I could tell you it probably had to do with family, and all of that, but I don't know specifically, so I wasn't thinking this, that, that, that and that, I wasn't counting them in my head, I just really tried to separate myself from the experience and just let whatever's going to pop up, pop up because I was afraid that if I was connected to it that I was going to affect the outcome.*

(Student I) So does that mean you can't name off the five items right now? They're still sort of in a vague … you dealt with them … *Yeah, it's sort of … I don't know specifically what they are, I do know specifically in the big picture what they add up to, but I don't know if I sat there and counted them they would add up to nine.*

Okay, your second wish was being able to have a relationship; eliminate the barriers. Can you identify those barriers consciously and tell me what they are? *Yeah, I feel like … extremely trapped when I get into a relationship, I just feel trapped. And I feel … what happens is I go inward, and I just stop being me. I feel like I'm losing myself and losing my freedom. And because I have a hard time confronting, or had a hard time confronting, I …*

Consciously, logically, rationally … are you trapped in that situation? Actually? *No.*

Centrum, … *I should close my eyes again.*

Centrum, are you willing to cooperate in resolving this relationship problem? YES

Step one, Centrum – I ask that you investigate it, investigate the roots, identify those parts of your mind that came into existence that still feel trapped and still cause you to feel that way. Then let me know with the word "complete" when you have done so. COMPLETE

Centrum, did you identify one or more such parts? YES

Centrum, how many such parts are there? How many experiences contributed to that? THREE

Centrum, in light of what I've been guiding you to do, do you, Centrum, know what to do without my assistance? YES

Please accomplish that task, and let me know when you have done so. COMPLETE

Were you successful with all three, Centrum? YES

Centrum, please follow up now, search to identify any remaining part or parts that might cause the problem to continue. COMPLETE

Did you identify any, Centrum? Any remaining parts? NO

Okay. Centrum, are you satisfied that that issue has now been completely resolved, and you are now free to have the kind of relationships that you consciously want to have. Are you satisfied, Centrum? YES

I might have asked if any part objected. Instead, I followed my intuition and continued.

Then Centrum, please provide that same level of conviction consciously, doing so by elevating all of the memories involved so that you can consciously comprehend the process by which that barrier became reality. Are you willing to do that, Centrum? YES

Let me know by the word "complete" when you have done so. COMPLETE

Back to you consciously now, Barbara. Are you satisfied with that one, or is there more you want to know? *I'm satisfied.*

I might have guided her to test completion by using her imagination.

Centrum, are you willing to address that third issue, the issue of your being able to have a satisfying sexual experience, as appropriate, so that sexual experience becomes a natural part of your life – fulfilling, joyful, all that it can be – Centrum, are you willing to cooperate in resolving any barrier to that experience? YES

The third goal.

Take the first step, Centrum. Investigate. This is a consequence of life experiences, look at them, identify those parts of your mind that came into existence in those conditions. And let me know when you have done so. COMPLETE

Centrum, how many such parts did you identify? FOUR

Okay. Four. And, Centrum, do you know what to do to fix this one? YES

I erred at this point. I failed to ask Centrum to search for additional parts.

Willing to do that now, Centrum? YES

Let me know when you have done so. COMPLETE

And Centrum, were you successful? YES

Then Centrum, please take the final step. Let there be full, complete, conscious comprehension. Let me know when you have done that. COMPLETE

And, back to you consciously, Barbara. Are you happy, satisfied? Is there more you want to know? *No.*

Then, at your own pace, Barbara, I ask that you rouse yourself. No hurry. If you want to stay there and think about it for a while, that's okay. What do you think? *I didn't have any recall of new memories, or anything like that. I don't know if I'm ready for that anyway.*

This surprised me. I had assumed she had the memories.

Oh, you didn't recall. That's okay. *Yeah, there's things that I recall that I could recall before, but no new memories to recall. So, maybe there's just a lot of communication that's going on at the subconscious level that I'm not consciously aware of. So …*

Well, we will open that door when we need to. Now, during the interim between now and when we meet, I encourage you – it's not homework you have to do

– but I really encourage you to write about this experience. *Okay, I can do that.*

I don't care if you burn it immediately after you write. Writing forces organization, mental compartmentalization. Puts a cap on things. *Okay.*

(Student A) How do you feel now? *Um … tired. (laughs) Maybe I'm just really relaxed, though. Curious to see how things are going to unfold for me.*

So where are you on that scale? *I'm like a two …*   **Referring to the anxiety scale.**

Still just a two? *Yeah, that's pretty good for me.*

Well, we're going to see if we can put a cap on that. Centrum, there's still some anxiety remaining. Centrum, is that anxiety serving useful purpose in your life now? YES

Centrum, is it protecting you in some way? YES

Centrum, please let there be conscious awareness of that purpose. Write it on the chalkboard, or communicate it to conscious some way. *"Nervous" … that's what came up on the chalkboard.*

The word nervous? Centrum, do you understand why you're nervous? YES

Would it be okay for you to know consciously why you're nervous? YES

Then let that be known, Centrum. *I think it's just being in front of all of these people …*

Centrum, is that accurate? A conscious opinion, what that accurate? *Yes. It wrote "people" on the board. (laughs)*

Okay, now, in your conscious opinion, Barbara, do you think there is any real justification for being nervous?

Or is that a product of your imagination in some way? *Yeah, I think it's just a product. There's really no reason to be nervous.*

Centrum, do you now agree with that? YES

Then Centrum, tell me, do you know how to eliminate that anxiety? Do you know what to do and how to do it? YES

Please let me know when you have done so. COMPLETE

Okay, Lady Barbara. How do you feel now? *I feel calm, I feel better.*

Better? Where are you on the zero to ten scale? Do you feel any anxiety at all? *No, I feel alright.*

Are you surprised you had the mental ability to just turn it off like that? Does that surprise you? *I think just becoming aware, and realizing that it's not really justified is a big part of it.*

Consciously, we theorize about these things. We know that there's no real, actual, justifiable reason … and yet there is. And when we really come to terms with it, like you just did, actually come to terms with it, there's no reason for it, it ceases to be. Okay? *Mm-hm.*

Class, do you have questions for her, or for me? Are all of you are now ready to take on a patient, and demonstrate your proficiency?

(Student) Well, you asked about two or three hundred questions here, I'm trying to write them down you know, following the … so, you know, I don't feel like I'm ready to do it. I could feel my way, but you had the right questions at the right time.

Did you have a question (points at student) or are you ready to go home?

(Student) Yeah, did you ever encounter patients that would resist the notion of Centrum? Or perhaps they want a different name for it, or …

Yes to both.

(Student) And how does that usually go?

If they resist the notion … uh, that this is too far off the wall, or hokey pokey, or whatever they might consider it – it rarely, rarely happens. Not once in a hundred patients, I don't think. Patients just follow this and love this. But in that situation, I say okay, we won't use this technique, and I will proceed with some other approach. Maybe age regression would work under hypnosis. Guide them through remembering the first time, and then progress from there. The ultimate objective is unconscious comprehension. That's where change happens. And approaching it by regressive work means that you're working through consciousness, as opposed to bypassing conscious resistance. Again, it doesn't happen often, but sometimes people don't like the idea of a chalkboard. They associate negative things with school, perhaps. They want to use a computer screen, or they want to use a white board, or they like green boards, or whatever else. I simply say to them, "I will no doubt slip and call your computer screen a chalkboard, but you know what I mean, don't you?"

(Student) I guess your process doesn't go into causal effects … it talks about those nine issues that she had, but you didn't really touch on any of them that much, and so I'm wondering, are you making the assumption that unconscious knows how, exactly how to 'fix' any of those issues. It seems like you're making an assumption that people know how to fix those problems.

In this situation, yes, I'm making that assumption, and I'm doing so on the basis of past successes. I may well sense, or the patient may blatantly confront me with "that doesn't make sense," "I didn't understand that," and Centrum is unable to explain that either. Well that's when I get involved, in a more traditional role as a therapist. If, for example, one of her points had been, "I was in that park, and that guy who came up to me, he touched me, and I now remember that, but I don't understand how that had any effect on me." Centrum, do you understand how that effect took place? Yes or no. If yes, then I ask Centrum to reach a conclusion. If no, then I get involved, I get some information in a traditional way, and then I put forth a possible explanation, and then inquire. Does that make sense consciously, does that make sense to you, Centrum?

(Student) So you don't believe that, I guess. It just makes me more curious than anything, I guess, to see the results.

Okay. Barbara and I will meet again, I hope, I expect, and any issues that she wants to deal with, we will deal with in a confidential setting. But I say to you, it's very reasonably possible that she has accomplished all three goals. I will obtain these questionnaires from her when I see her again, and I will show them to you. The before, and the after. *It's basically just re-educating the subconscious mind of the fact that the reasoning of those problems no longer exists, now.*

You've got it! *So it's not necessary now to retrieve those memories to a conscious state, or to understand why, consciously, that subconsciously you're re-educating the subconscious mind that it's not applicable anymore to be continuing those behaviors.*

Very nicely expressed.

(Student) Did I get that to mean that there's not so much a knowledge of specifics, there's sort of a blanket thing, whatever happened then doesn't apply now, so I can just sever connection with it. Is that sort of what you were saying? *Not really sever connection. Well, just to realize that being anxious anymore doesn't apply.*

(Student) So there's not, there's not some specific, you don't have to get into specifics of that, but there's some sort of blanket over that. *I think it's at a subconscious level, I'm not really aware of why when I'm feeling anxious, so I don't have to be aware of why it happened in the first place. Just that it's happening, and so then you re-educate it that it's not applicable in the present moment anymore, to respond that way, I guess.*

(Student) An unrelated question, I guess – When Centrum was doing the re-education of the nine parts, were you aware of the negotiations or was that all done in the blank, or … ? *I wasn't really aware of it, I was just trying not to get involved. I'm so left-minded that I'll just run myself in circles trying to think of stuff, or I'll try to figure it out.*

(Student) So you weren't aware of any negotiations? *No. I was just concentrating on the chalkboard and doing my best to just turn everything else off, and to just let Centrum and the subconscious or whatever just do whatever.*

I think probably most of the time, that's the way it happens. But, a significant number of times, the patient does have some awareness of that process taking place. And they usually have difficulty articulating it.

(Student) Just a couple questions. Um, why would you ask Centrum to bring things into consciousness? Why is that …?

Why do I?

(Student) Yeah.

Well, it's not because I think it's essential. I have difficulty in articulating a reasonable answer to that. I guess my subjective experience, over many times, tells me that somehow it's reinforcing. Somehow there's conscious satisfaction of completion that's valuable. And it is not necessary.

(Student) Okay. And I'm a little bit confused because I think of an unconscious Centrum, so it sounds like it all complies with the conscious …

I don't follow you.

(Student) Well, when you say, how can Centrum bring it into consciousness if it's still conscious when Centrum is unconscious?

How does it happen?

(Student) Yeah, how can it do that if it is unconscious?

Is that a sort of academic question; what is the mechanism that allows that communication?

(Student) No, no, no, I'm just thinking conscious, unconscious, so how can this consciousness be unconscious?

By communication.

(Student) With itself?

Please, answer it (points to another student).

(Student) Well, I'm just gonna say, how does anything unconscious become conscious? For example, you're not conscious of the fact that you're touching your fingers right now, but you are. It's a bad example, but …

I believe that kind of communication, and it is, as I understand it, communication, takes place through the senses. Through our senses. It's like the example, how do you spell cat? Half of the class sees the letters, and half the class hears the letters. It's through the senses that the information is communicated. Maybe by memory, by … I don't have an adequate answer to that question, you got a better one? (laughs) Got one I can answer?

(Student) Okay, okay, another thing, you talked about 'parts', and I'm familiar with parts and it seems like parts are really bad events in the past. Is that the same thing?

In my comprehension here, in this module of the mind, a 'part' is a name that represents that influence that is the consequence of an event, either good or bad.

(Student) Okay, so it's not an event.

It represents the consequence.

(Student) I thought it was really the way that you guys articulated everything that happened, that everything in the past that happened doesn't have to control us. I thought that was really interesting how she articulated it, and maybe it's a little critical if we haven't had her experiences, so I'm interested to know, had you thought about it before in those terms? It was very clear, and concise, and very logical how you articulated it.

For the benefit of the tape, the question is, has she been thinking about all of this? She has been able to articulate all of these events that have taken place during our session, has she been thinking about it? How is it that she can articulate that? *No, I hadn't really ever thought about that before, really. Um, but it all just makes sense for whatever reason, now. I don't know, going through that process of not having certain memories just pop up or just being able to differentiate just allowing the process to happen, and understanding, like how he put me through the process of finding those areas; finding and re-educating those areas, and then feeling calm now, it's very interesting. To not have to pick through everything consciously. I don't have to know why, it just seems to make sense. Yeah, it's interesting.*

(Student) I'm also struck by that idea, it seems to be whatever … I don't have to be concerned about the cause. It came up earlier in life, it doesn't concern me anymore. It's irrelevant. And life is much better with the present thinking. And you know it's an annoyance to deal with the early memories, you're sticking with what you know now. Maybe I'm reading too much into it, did that make sense or no? *It made sense, yeah. And I'm not necessarily … I think because my unconscious was kicking up all of this anxiety, the unconscious can be re-educated not to kick up any more, so I can … yeah, so, that was my main concern that I was going to get to involved in the whys and hows and I was afraid I wasn't going to be able to allow the process to happen, because my mind typically tends to get in the way; I'm always rationalizing, thinking, picking things apart, analyzing, so just to be able to turn that off and say I don't even have to do that, I can just let the subconscious take care of it, and just listening to him, reading the board, and whatever pops up pops up and not reading into it was freeing, it was really freeing to not have to pick it apart. What if I'm thinking the wrong thing, what if I'm interpreting it right, well, it doesn't even matter because subconsciously it's all happening, so I don't really have to understand or know, or remember for that fact, I may not even want to.*

(Student) I just got an image now, of jettisoning, a rocket jettisons the spent thing. So it's a several stage rocket, it's just jettisoning the spent fuel compartment that you used, and you're just able to fly in the present. I'm kind of fascinated by the mechanism.

Okay, do you have anything else you want to bring up,
or ask about?

I'm good

Della – Detecting Conscious Opinion Expressed as Communication from Centrum

Della was a 28-year-old female who presented with multiple
issues, the most important of which was her strongly jealous
nature. She was married, with two children, and the marriage
was in serious trouble, largely because of her jealousy.

The following excerpt from the beginning of this case is presented
in illustration of the too-often encountered problem of the patient
responding to questions that were directed to Centrum with conscious opinions about what the answers *should* be. Della had read
my introductory book (Yager, 1985), and responded to my questions in a way that convinced me she understood the concepts.

SECOND SESSION

Centrum, please indicate your willingness to communicate with me by this means by writing the word
"yes" on the chalkboard. YES

The chalkboard disappeared.

Centrum, are you willing to cooperate, to do some
work as I guide you and teach you how, to accomplish
your conscious goal? (No response)

Centrum, are you aware of your conscious concern
about your jealous nature? YES Centrum do you agree
that your jealousy is a problem? YES

Centrum, are you willing to cooperate, to do some
work as I guide you and teach you how, to accomplish
your conscious goal? YES

The "yes" response, followed immediately by the disappearance of the chalkboard, was unusual. This, followed by a "no" response to a question that is consistently responded to with a "yes" was my first clue that something was not right.

The three consistent "yes" answers, to questions where a "yes" answer would reasonably be expected, was misleadingly reassuring that the answers came from Centrum.

Centrum, are you capable of remembering events in your life? NO Centrum, are you capable of remembering the day you were married? YES

Centrum, are you capable of remembering her 20th birthday? NO

Centrum, are you intelligent? YES

Centrum, are you capable of communicating with other parts of your mind? NO

Centrum, does the model, the theory of Subliminal Therapy, make sense to you? NO Centrum, are you listening as we discuss how the unconscious domain seems to me to be made up of the many parts that represent influences you have learned in the course of living? YES Centrum, are you open to the possibility that that model may be accurate? YES

Centrum, please identify one of those parts of your mind that cause you to be jealous. Centrum, is my request clear to you? YES

Centrum, how old were you when you first experienced feeling jealous? (No response)

Inconsistency in the following three answers was my clue to challenge the source of the answers. Centrum can consistently be expected to remember events not available to consciousness.

The unexpected and the inconsistent nature of the answers to the succeeding questions were further clues that the answers were not coming from Centrum.

This "no" answer, in particular, was inconsistent since there had been a series of questions and answers that had flowed in a normal way.

Additionally, the overall flow of the process simply did not 'feel' right.

Gentle confrontational discussion at this juncture confirmed that Della had been responding with her conscious opinion in lieu of responses on the chalkboard. *I think I try too hard.*

Della was requested to enter trance on her own, which she did, and the trance was deepened by the Three Candle technique described in my book (Yager, 2008). She was then taught to use ideo-motor (finger) responses rather than the chalkboard and her jealousy problem was successfully resolved.

Tom – A Case of Pain from a Spinal Cord Injury

Tom was a 60-year-old male who suffered spinal cord injury at age 22 in an automobile accident. He has been wheelchair-bound since the accident, and reported pain from cramping of muscles in his legs and lower back since the accident. He reported, *"When I try to stop it at night, it gains control. That's the worst time. Now I'm working on my 'pain about the pain' and the anxiety that causes."*

Eight sessions were involved, following the initial history-taking session, and the following excerpts are quoted. The concept of Centrum as a higher self (*"beyond our thinking"*) was familiar to him from other experiences. He was taught self-hypnosis in the first session and reported its consistent use afterward. Only excerpts are provided in this case report; however, the flow of treatment should be evident.

SESSION 2

Centrum, do you believe you now understand all aspects of the pain problem? Is the picture clear to you? PICTURE IS CLEAR Centrum, is one or more parts of your mind actively causing or exacerbating the pain? YES Centrum how many parts are acting that way? THREE Centrum, are you in communication with all three of those parts? YES

The "Picture is Clear" response was unusual, and caused me to consider the possibility of conscious response; however, the way it was orally stated was reassuring, therefore I went ahead.

Centrum, please select one of those parts and proceed in this way: First, listen to the part. Learn what you need to know in order to be able to educate the part about your present life situation and life conditions. Centrum, is that clear to you? Is my request clear to you? YES Then Centrum, please accomplish that task and let me know when you have done so. COMPLETE Centrum were you successful in persuading that part to your way of thinking? YES

Centrum, would it be okay for you to know consciously, for you to consciously understand the work you just accomplished? YES Centrum, please elevate that understanding to consciousness. Let the memory of the event become conscious, together with the understanding of the effect of that event on your life today. COMPLETE Tom, does that make sense to you consciously? Does it satisfy your need to know? *Yes.*

Centrum, please repeat the same protocol with the second of the three parts. First, listen, then educate the part. Persuade the part to your way of thinking and let me know by the word "complete" when you have completed the task. COMPLETE Centrum, were you successful? YES

Centrum, please repeat that procedure with the third of those three parts. Listen, then educate, and let me know when you have completed the task. COMPLETE Centrum were you successful? YES Centrum please elevate the understanding of those last two parts to conscious awareness, as you did in the first case. COMPLETE Tom, do both of those issues make sense to you consciously? *Yes.*

Centrum, because it is so commonly true that identifying and resolving one issue makes it possible, and only then possible, to identify another, I ask that you again search to identify any remaining part, that for any reason whatsoever, might contribute to the pain problem. Let me know when you've completed the search by the word "complete". COMPLETE Centrum, did you identify any remaining part? YES How many did you identify? ONE Centrum, are you in communication with that part? YES Do you know what to do without further assistance from me? YES Then please accomplish that task, listen, then educate. Let me know by the word "complete" when you have done so. COMPLETE Centrum, were you successful? YES Then Centrum, please elevate that awareness, that understanding, to consciousness. COMPLETE Tom, does all of that make sense? *Yes.*

Note this recurring request, and the fact that additional parts are consistently identified. I have not conceived of a satisfying explanation for this, other than the explanation afforded Centrum; nevertheless, the effect is consistent.

Centrum, yet again I ask that you reinvestigate, that you search to identify any remaining part of your mind that might cause the pain to continue. COMPLETE Centrum, did you identify any remaining part? YES How many? ONE Centrum, do you know what to do? YES Centrum, please do what you need to do. COMPLETE Were you successful? YES

Centrum, yet again, please search to identify any remaining part. COMPLETE Centrum, did you identify any remaining part? NO

Centrum, is it advisable that you eliminate all discomfort, all pain? YES Centrum, are you now capable of accomplishing that without assistance from me? YES Are you willing to do that now? YES Then Centrum, please do so. Tom, please advise me when you are at zero. *Woo hoo!*

Tom's response was apparently an expression of amazement. Even in trance, he was smiling.

Centrum is there anything more to be done at this point? Is there any remaining, perhaps peripheral, issue in need of attention? NO Tom, if you will please, at your own pace, rouse yourself from trance and let's discuss what just happened.

I feel good. It all made good sense. It was nice to have a guide.

Tom, can you articulate the five issues that Centrum just resolved?

#1 was my refusal to have my leg cut off.

#2 was when I was wounded in the leg. I had to wait. There was no medical attention available.

#3 was when I was a bit by a dog at around my 17th or 18th year.

#4 I had to kill an animal that had been injured.

#5 was erasing all of the pictures.

Centrum, do you believe it's possible, however remote, to re-establish neural connection with the muscles of your leg, to improve their condition? YES Centrum please investigate the possibility between now and the next time we meet. Take advantage of any and all inputs and insights that might assist you. Are you willing to do that? YES

Although some of these responses were not fully understood by me, they were apparently understood by him – and that's all that matters. In employing ST, the therapist is more divorced from content than with other therapeutic techniques.

SESSION 3

Tom reported a pain level of five (on the zero to ten scale) while in transit to the office for our session. He also reported being (now) at level one, which he said was typical of what happened when he comes here. He reported having had two good days, although not consecutive days, since the last session, in addition to today. *Now I am even more determined.*

Tom, have you continued to practice self-hypnosis? *Yes, I have. I do it every night and a sharp pain in my leg will bring me out of the state. I am successful in relieving the pain if I can feel it coming on, or if it's mild. I'm getting better at it. Last night I asked Centrum to eliminate needless pain. I woke up feeling much better, alive, more energy, and very little pain. The worst of all times is when I have to sit on the john, or if I'm going up a hill in my wheelchair.*

Centrum, are you willing to continue this work? YES Centrum, please investigate the situation, reviewing what you did before. Re-evaluate that work in the light of what has happened and what you have learned this week. OKAY Centrum, did you identify any other part of your mind, any other influence in need of attention? MAYBE Centrum, please concentrate on that issue. Determine whether or not it exists. IT EXISTS Centrum, is it represented by some part of your mind? NO Centrum what is it? A BLACK MASS THAT HOVERS ABOUT MY RIGHT LEG

The responses from Centrum from this point onward were more elaborate than previously. I suspected conscious responses, but was assured by Tom that they were on his chalkboard.

Centrum, do you understand the nature of that black mass, or the origin of it? NO Centrum, please search to identify any part of your mind that does understand its nature and origin. COMPLETE Centrum, did you identify such a part? ENERGY PUSHING EACH OTHER. ENERGY AGAINST ENERGY. I DON'T KNOW WHAT CAUSED IT

Centrum, does the black mass represent anything? NO BEING ABLE TO CHANGE, OR SOMETHING Centrum, what are those two energies that push against each other? IT HAD SOMETHING TO DO WITH ... IN ORDER TO MOVE IT HURTS, AND I DON'T WANT TO HURT, SO I'M PUSHING AGAINST THE ENERGY. PUSHING BACK AGAINST IT SO IT DOESN'T MOVE. Tom, does all of that makes sense to you? *Yes.*

Centrum, is it possible for you to move without hurting? YES Centrum, do you know how to make that happen? YES Are you willing to do so? YES Centrum, please do all you know to erase that black mass. COMPLETE Centrum, please elevate to consciousness full understanding of the work you just did.

It was effort and counter-effort. The fear was of feeling pain. Washed it away. It's very relaxed now.

Centrum, is the black mass there now? NO, ONLY THE THOUGHT IT MIGHT RETURN

Centrum, please investigate the possibility that it might return. Is my request clear to you? YES Then please do so. OKAY Centrum, did you identify any part of your mind, any issues in need of attention? YES, ONE Centrum do you know what to do at this point? YES Let me know when you have done. OKAY Centrum, were you successful? I BELIEVE SO Centrum, please let there be conscious understanding of the work you just did. Centrum is there any

You might have proceeded differently than me at this point. And yours might well have been more effective than mine.

There were occasions such as this when there were no responses from Centrum before there was a conscious response from Tom. This is not usual, but on the other hand, it is not unusual.

Note that Centrum is anticipating the next question, answering before being asked in responding "YES, ONE."

additional task apparent to you? NO Tom, are you at this point completely comfortable? *Yes.*

Centrum, do you consider the possibility of re-establishing neural connection as I requested of you? NO Centrum, do you still believe it may be possible? I DON'T KNOW Centrum, are you willing to pursue that, to investigate? YES Then please do so. COMPLETE Centrum, do you consider this possibility worth pursuing? I DON'T KNOW Centrum, would anything be lost by doing so? NO

I might have ended the session at this point; however, we had previously discussed different, possible ways to eliminate the pain. This one was well-founded and in proceeding, I was acting on instinct.

At this point, I delivered a mini-lecture on the power of our imagination, which I believe to be the single most powerful means at our disposal, to change the way we experience life, suggesting that he practice imaging what he desired as a homework assignment.

SESSION 4

Tom reported that at night pain builds up on one side and wakes him up. He then turns over and goes back to sleep. This happens every forty minutes to two hours. He reported that until last week he was able to experience deep sleep. *I need to regenerate that experience.*

Sleep issues had not previously been mentioned, so I elected to pursue this avenue of inquiry.

Centrum, are you aware of this sleep issue and the problem it creates? YES Centrum, are you willing to address this issue? YES Then Centrum, please investigate, find out what is happening and why. COMPLETE Centrum, do you believe you now understand the cause and effect of this problem? Is the picture clear to you? YES

Centrum, please identify those parts that are causing the problem. There's a part that is reacting to something, a part that is not always engaged. IF I'M HAVING FUN, OR FOCUSED, IT DOES NOT REACT. IF I'M FOCUSED ON CONSEQUENCE, I REACT VIA THE PAIN

Again, the content is not understood by me, yet the process continues smoothly. If I had considered it necessary to have understood consciously, I could have interrupted the flow and asked questions.

Centrum, do you see a solution to this problem? For example, is it possible for that controlling part to maintain comfort? YES, IT'S IN WHEN I'M HAVING FUN Centrum, does that seem to be a realistic solution to you? YES Centrum, are you capable of making that happen? YES Are you willing to do that now? YES Then Centrum, please do so. COMPLETE Centrum, please reinvestigate this issue. Identify any other parts of your mind, any other issues in need of attention. COMPLETE Centrum, did you identify any? YES, FIVE

Centrum, do you need assistance in resolving those issues you have identified? NO Then please accomplish that task. COMPLETE Centrum, were you successful with all five? YES

I can feel myself going into a deep sleep.

Centrum, please reinvestigate. Identify any other issue, any other part of your mind, in need of attention. COMPLETE Did you identify any? NO

My imagery is vibrational energy. It's like an electric rain in my back at the injury. Then I can get warm energy back to that area.

Centrum, I believe you have the requisite abilities to accomplish the regeneration of tissue, and I want to know if you are willing to investigate this possibility. YES Then Centrum, please do so. FOUR MONTHS

Centrum, what are you saying? HEALING CAN HAPPEN IN FOUR MONTHS Centrum, are you capable of making that happen? YES Centrum, please take whatever steps you need to take, doing so now. OKAY Centrum, are there any other peripheral issues? NO Centrum, does any other subject need to be put on the table? NO

> Once the protocol has been learned, and the direction of work to be accomplished has been defined, the clinician is advised to step out of the way and allow the work to be completed.

> In this situation, I was at a loss to logically define the next step to take. My question was an act of instinct.

Tom, if you will please, at your own pace and after visualizing that vibratory energy doing its work, please rouse yourself.

My body was heavy with energy. It was like being in a deep sleep physically.

SESSION 5

Tom reported: *I have pain, but somehow I'm more focused and less dispersed. When the pain comes it passes, it doesn't stay. I don't have the anxiety I had. The pain was not as bad during the recent cold, wet weather as it has been in the past. I'm continuing to communicate with Centrum. I put him to work every night. I have been picturing myself sending in white light to areas that were damaged.*

I am always pleased by reports of the patient having had direct communication with Centrum. Although I consistently recommend and encourage such interaction, patients seldom report having done so.

Centrum, you're doing great! Thank you. Centrum, is there anything yet to be done to further ease the pain, anything that you are aware of? MAYBE Then Centrum, please investigate this possibility. COMPLETE Centrum, did you identify any other influence or part of your mind in need of attention? YES

Centrum, are you willing that there be conscious awareness of the issues?

I get the feeling that it's about raising consciousness. If I raise my consciousness, Centrum can do more work.

Sometimes expressions of conscious opinion can lead you down the wrong path, yet they may be communications from Centrum. To check, ask Centrum.

Centrum, is that accurate? YES

I think I know how to do this. It means to get awareness that the mind and body are one.

Centrum, is that accurate? YES

As long as I separate the two, and I have been, it causes this block.

Centrum, I don't understand what's going on. Do you know how to resolve this issue? YES Then Centrum, please do so. COMPLETE Centrum were you successful? YES

Tom, are you aware of any difference in your experience?

I think so. It's like role playing, and I can drop the role play. Something happened.

Centrum, is there anything more regarding that issue, anything more to be done? NO

Centrum are you willing to explore the possibility that that 'black energy' can, in some way, be healed? YES Then Centrum, please do that between now and the next time we meet.

SESSION 6

Tom reported that he had been able to reduce the morphine level in the pain pump he had been using. *My intestines have recovered, I hear those stomach noises again.* He also reported having begun to use a new medication, Lyrica, which seemed to be effective. I suggested that he design an imagery program focused on gaining physical control. This was discussed and no other issues came up this session.

SESSION 7

Tom reported continually lowering the medication level, especially morphine, although his legs had been in almost constant cramped condition. *It's harder for me to be in trance when my legs hurt, like now.*

Centrum are you willing to investigate the possibility that you can intervene in some helpful way? YES Then Centrum, please do whatever it is possible for you to do. COMPLETE Centrum, as another possible way, interrupt the neural communication between your legs and your brain. Please investigate the possibility, and if it is possible, make it happen. OKAY

At this point I introduced Tom to the concept of using his 'sanctuary'. I guided him to create his imagined sanctuary while in trance, and to occupy that sanctuary. For elaboration on this technique, see my book (Yager, 2008).

This is my place where it's okay not to feel pain all the time. I can feel comfortable.

Tom, you can return to your sanctuary as often as you wish, and stay there as long as you wish while you heal, and you can continue in comfort even when it's time to leave the sanctuary, perhaps to attend to some necessary issue. And even then, you bring back with you the benefits of the sanctuary, and continue to enjoy those benefits.

Tom, if you will please, leave your sanctuary, now, returning to this place, here with me, bringing with you the comfort and peace of mind you experienced in the sanctuary.

SESSION 8

Tom reported that during the last session he got so deep in trance he was pain-free for four days. *It was concrete. Something really happened. Centrum's actions were the effect on the development. Centrum seemed to me to be doing something to affect the development of the relief.*

Centrum, we want to know what works. Maybe just hypnotic depth worked last time, but maybe it was what you did. Centrum, was it what you did that made the difference? YES

Centrum, is it possible for you to be pain free on a continual basis? YES Centrum, please support that goal, not just here and now, but in the days, weeks and months ahead.

Requests to Centrum for continued work between sessions are not usually carried out. I have no explanation for this.

Something was happening. Centrum just did something.

In follow-up phone calls one week and then one month later, Tom reported continuing pain, but at a greatly reduced level than when he began the work with me. He is now able to sleep adequately and to return to work – an important issue for him.

Cindy – Unusual Resolution of Anger

Cindy was a 23-year-old graduate student with a bad case of subconsciously inspired and inappropriate anger that interfered with her life in multiple ways. She was attractive, quick-witted and displayed a great deal of charm, yet she had difficulty maintaining relationships with males and females alike; they were simply not willing to deal with the overt display of anger focused on any issue that did not go just as she wanted. The anger had been problematic since before high school.

Cindy saw me on only two occasions before she was forced by unexpected financial reasons to return home to a Midwestern city. Our work was not complete, yet in a telephone conversations many weeks later, she reported experiencing much less anger, especially in social situations. She had read the introductory book and had practiced self-hypnosis daily. The stage had been set for employing ST, Centrum was willing to cooperate, and she was optimistic about the outcome.

SECOND SESSION

Centrum, are you aware of your conscious concern about the excessive anger? YES Centrum, are you also concerned about that excessive anger? NO Centrum are you willing to cooperate, to do some work as I

Initially expressed lack of concern on the part of Centrum is not unusual.

guide you and teach you how, with the objective of possibly eliminating the excessive anger? NOT YET

Centrum, do you believe the anger serves a useful purpose in your life? YES NO Centrum, do you believe it is in your best interest to continue to experience that anger? YES NO

I am probing for a way to get my 'foot in the door.' I am searching to identify common ground from which I can lead Centrum to explore other possibilities.

Centrum, I wonder if you were attentive as you read the book on ST, because I wonder if the model of the mind portrayed there seems accurate and sensible to you. Does it seem so? YES

Centrum, when you were a little girl the exaggerated anger was understandable and appropriate in some situations. However, Centrum, that exaggerated reaction is no longer appropriate; it makes no sense in your adult life. Are you willing to consider whether or not this anger has value in your life now? NO

Having found that common issue (Centrum agreed the model of ST makes sense), I now go down that road.

Cindy, please explain, aloud, the reasons you want to eliminate the excessive anger from your life. In doing so, you will be explaining the situation to Centrum.

Not feeling angry will make me feel better. It will improve my relationships and I can be the kind of person I want to be. Life will be more peaceful.

It is highly important that the clinician rely on the opinions, values and beliefs of the patient, rather than lecturing on the reasons for change that are apparent to the clinician.

Centrum, does the concept of 'parts' make sense to you? NO Centrum, does the concept of reconditioning by re-education make sense to you? I am referring to the concept of identifying and educating the different parts of your mind about your present life situation, needs and values. Does this concept make sense to you? YES

My previous question about Centrum's understanding was not comprehensive enough; it did not ask about 'parts'.

Centrum, do you believe you have the ability to remember and examine the experiences in your life and to understand those experiences in the light of present knowledge? YES

Rather than take the time for explanation about 'parts', I decided to pursue a different avenue.

Centrum, please examine the first experience you can identify in which anger was the dominant influence at the time. Is it apparent to you how anger was affecting you in that situation? YES Centrum, is that same reaction appropriate in your life as an adult? NO

Centrum, please examine and evaluate the next experience that you can identify in which anger was the dominant force. COMPLETE Centrum, is the influence of that experience clear to you? YES Centrum, is that reaction appropriate now in your life as an adult? NO

The identification and resolution of these parts was the basic objective of this work; therefore the different avenue begun above was effective. However, it could have failed, in which case I would have returned to educate Centrum about 'parts'.

Centrum, I ask that you repeat this examination of early influences, identifying and evaluating every influence, every part of your mind, evaluating the appropriateness of their influence in current life. COMPLETE Centrum, is the effect of all those experiences clear to you now? YES Centrum, are any of those lessons or influences appropriate in your life now? SOME, NO

Cindy, please rouse yourself from trance and let's discuss this experience. The test of success in using ST lies in the real world. You may have achieved that success, or you may not; however, I want it to be clear to you that if the anger surfaces again, it does not mean this work has been unsuccessful, it simply means that it is incomplete. We will complete it as we continue the work we have begun.

Some benefit of this work was reported during our previously mentioned telephone conversation; however, it was apparent to me at this time that the work was not complete. There remained one or more parts, yet to be identified, that continued to cause the experiences of anger.

Suzi – The Resolution of Alcohol Abuse

Suzi was a 47-year-old female who presented with problems of insomnia, agoraphobia and alcohol abuse. For unknown reasons, Suzi withdrew from treatment following her second session. There is, therefore, no measure of the success of the treatments employed; however, the flow of the second session indicated optimism for its outcome. The second session was a two-hour session and the insomnia problem was addressed first without a clear, satisfactory conclusion. On the other hand, the following, excerpted portion addressing her alcohol abuse problem, seemed to indicate a favorable outcome.

SESSION TWO

Centrum, are you aware of your conscious concern about your desire for alcohol? YES Centrum, are you willing to cooperate, to do some work as I guide you and teach you how, with the objective of eliminating that desire for alcohol? YES

Centrum, please investigate the roots of your desire for alcohol, doing so either with or without conscious awareness, as you deem appropriate. Centrum, is that request clear to you? YES Then Centrum, please accomplish that task and let me know when you have completed it. COMPLETE Centrum, do you believe you now understand how you developed that excessive desire for alcohol? YES

Giving Centrum the okay to investigate without conscious awareness can preclude unconscious interference due to objection to there being conscious awareness. This 'permission' may not be necessary, but nothing is lost by including it.

Centrum, please identify that part, or those parts as the case may be, of your mind that are responsible for the continuation of this desire for alcohol, even though it is inappropriate in your present life. COMPLETE Centrum, did you identify one or more such parts? YES How many? ONE Centrum, are you in communication with that part? YES Then Centrum, please repeat the protocol you have been using previously today. Let me know when that task is complete. COMPLETE Centrum, were you successful? I THINK SO

Centrum, does that part still desire to drink in some situations? YES Centrum, do you know what that situation is? YES Centrum, do you agree with the position that part is taking in affirming the need in some situation where it would be appropriate to experience that desire? NO Then Centrum, please communicate further with that part. Ensure that you understand the position and beliefs of that part so that you can effectively persuade that part to your way of thinking. IT'S A TRICKY PART, IT WANTS TO COMPROMISE

> The hesitant, "I think so" response to the previous question prompted me to pursue a more definitive answer.

Centrum, do you understand why it wants to compromise? (No response)

Centrum, do you agree that compromise is the best solution to this problem? NO Centrum, please communicate even further with that part, convince that part that it is in the best interest of all that you eliminate that excessive drive for alcohol.

> Lack of response to this question prompted me to be creative. I sought clarification of Centrum's position and assumed that Centrum was capable of handling the situation.

I can't read the word, it's jumbled.

Centrum, is some other part of your mind also involved, interfering with this work? YES Centrum, please establish communication with this interfering part and do all you can do to persuade it to cease interfering. IT'S A BATTLE Centrum, are you winning the battle? YES

> This question was based on my experience, rather than being logically derived. Interference from an objecting, interfering part that has not yet been identified is a common situation in employing ST.

Centrum, please continue this work, keeping in mind that all parts are well-intended, even this interfering part, and that it is your task to provide the reconditioning required to change the position held by the part.

The chalkboard is jumbled again.

Centrum, some part is interfering with this work, doing so by jumbling the answers. Perhaps this is a new part. Do you understand your task in resolving this problem? YES Centrum are you willing to

> This verbatim transcript revealed that I had not chosen the best language to use.

continue this work? YES Then please do so, let me know when the work is complete. (No response during a full two-minute silence)

Centrum, did you complete the task of resolving the interfering influence? YES Centrum, are all parts now willing to support your conscious needs and goals? YES Centrum, please elevate to consciousness full and complete understanding of the work you just did. COMPLETE

Again, I failed to use the best phrasing, and yet Centrum was able to handle the situation, taking the necessary steps to complete the work.

Suzi, does the information make sense to you? Does it satisfy your conscious need to understand how you learned to want to drink? *Yes.*

Could you, if I requested it, articulate the reasons and the means whereby you learned to desire alcohol in an excessive way? *Yes.*

Normally, if she was willing, I would have asked her to recount the details. In this case, the treatment hour was approaching the end.

Centrum, just to be sure, I again ask that you search the far reaches of your mind to identify any part of your mind that has in the past, or might in the future, cause the experience of the excessive desire for alcohol. OKAY Centrum, did you identify any remaining parts? NO Thank you Centrum. Great work!

Suzi, if you will please now, rouse yourself from trance.

That was something! My mind kept telling me, "You're not in the same trance you were before." I felt like I was deeper in trance. Was that two hours? That's crazy!

Pete – Excerpts from a Case of Panic Attacks

Pete was a 39-year-old male who presented with two basic issues. The following transcription followed resolution of one issue, panic attacks, and is presented here to illustrate treatment of that disorder.

Centrum, are you willing to continue this work with the objective of eliminating the panic attacks? YES Centrum, please investigate this problem. Find out how, why, when and where you learned to experience panic attacks. Centrum, is my request clear to you? YES Then please conduct that investigation and identify any parts of your mind that are actively causing you to experience panic attacks. COMPLETE Centrum, did you identify any such parts? YES How many? ONE

Centrum, please repeat the protocol used in the previous work. First listen, then educate that part about present reality. COMPLETE Centrum, were you successful? YES

Centrum, do you already have full conscious memory of the event you just uncovered? YES

Pete, are you satisfied with your understanding of how that event has affected your life? *No.*

It would have been irrational to have asked Pete if he had full understanding at a conscious level. Even so, the answer received was not an accurate answer.

Centrum, please elevate that memory, together with the understanding of how that event has affected you since that time. COMPLETE Pete, are you now satisfied? *Yes.*

Centrum, please search to identify any remaining part of your mind that might still be acting in a way to cause panic attacks to continue. COMPLETE Did you identify any parts? YES How many? FOUR Centrum, do you know what to do? YES Then Centrum, please accomplish that task. Listen and then educate, and let me know by the word "complete" when you have done so. COMPLETE Centrum, were you successful with resolving all four of those issues? YES Centrum, please elevate to consciousness the memory of those experiences, together with the understanding of the influence of each of those four events. COMPLETE

There is value in obtaining conscious memories and understanding of those memories; however, it seems not to be essential.

Pete, are you satisfied with your understanding of all four of those issues? *Yes.*

Centrum, please search further to identify any remaining part that was not uncovered previously. COMPLETE Centrum, did you identify any such parts? YES, TWO Centrum, you know what to do, please resolve those two issues. COMPLETE Centrum, were you successful with both of those issues? YES Centrum, please elevate to consciousness the memories and understanding of those two issues. COMPLETE

Pete, are you satisfied with your understanding of both of those issues? *Yes.*

Centrum, please search yet again to identify any remaining parts. COMPLETE Did you identify any such parts? YES, ONE Centrum, please do your work as you know how. Let me know when you have done so. COMPLETE Centrum, were you successful in resolving that issue? YES Once again Centrum, I ask that you search. As is so often true, as you have already demonstrated, when one issue is resolved it then, and only then, becomes possible to identify another. See if there is another part. COMPLETE Did you identify any? NO

Pete, are you satisfied with that one? *Yes.*

Thank you Centrum. Great work!

Pete, if you will please, rouse yourself from trance. Does the whole picture now seem complete to you? If I ask you to do so, would you be able to describe the process by which you learned to experience those panic attacks? *Yes.* Do you believe the panic attacks will continue? *It's hard to believe the show is over.*

Centrum, do you believe the show is over? YES

At the conclusion of one week, and at follow-up, Pete reported no further panic attacks.

Lorrie – A Case of Dry Eyes

Lorrie, a 40-year-old female, had experienced laser surgery on both eyes six years ago and had experienced constant dry eyes since then. She had taken Restasis (which causes the eyes to generate tears) successfully for four years, interrupting the med in preparation for pregnancy. When the medication was resumed, only modest benefit resulted. She had tried acupuncture and other treatments without improvement, reporting that when she cries, there are no tears. Lorrie had not read the introductory book before our second meeting and so it was necessary to verbally introduce ST. The agreed-upon goal of our work was to restore tearing, possibly by re-establishing the necessary neural communication. This excerpted section from our meetings turned out to have been almost the complete resolution; only one additional part was identified.

SECOND SESSION

Lorrie, you are not off the hook; I still encourage you to read my little book. In the meantime, however, let me introduce you to this technique that I call ST, so that we can begin work today. Subliminal Therapy is based on certain assumptions, the first of which is that our mentality is in part conscious, but in much greater part unconscious. Moreover, the unconscious domain seems to be made up of the accumulation of influences from life experiences. I refer to these influences as 'parts', for lack of a better word. We seem also to have a higher level of mental functioning there in the unconscious domain. I refer to this level of functioning as Centrum, and I will be guiding Centrum to do the work of therapy. In other words, I will be communicating with Centrum, offering guidance and perhaps information as Centrum does the actual work of therapy. To do this, I must be able to communicate

This is a typical narration I use in situations where the patient has not had previous exposure to ST and has not read the introductory book.

with Centrum, and that is where you come in at a conscious level of awareness. As we do this work together, it will be your job, consciously, to create an image of a chalkboard upon which Centrum can write, and then to report to me what Centrum has written. I cannot see your chalkboard and it is, therefore, exceedingly important that you reliably and accurately tell me what Centrum has written. You see, Lorrie, the chalkboard becomes a way of differentiating between the communications from Centrum and your conscious opinions about what should be written.

Let's begin this way. Lorrie, please create a mental image of a chalkboard there in your mind's eye. Let me know when you have that image clearly established. *I have it.* Centrum, please write the word "yes" in indication of willingness to communicate in this way. YES Now, Lorrie, you might well be thinking something like, "Well, it says 'yes', but how do I know if I didn't just think that up and write it there? How do I know that came from Centrum?" That would certainly be a valid question. Let me answer it this way. Centrum, please the erase word "yes" and replace it with a different word. This time, Centrum, please select a word that will surprise you consciously, some word that you will know you didn't think up and put there. Please write that word now. DON'T

Lorrie, are you satisfied you did not consciously write that word on the chalkboard? *Yes.*

Centrum, are you aware of your conscious concern about the dry eyes and about the problems they create in your life? NO, I'M NOT Lorrie, please explain. Express in your own words how the dry eyes impact your life.

They are often painful. They are embarrassing in social situations, and they interfere with my ability to work. I am constantly distressed and anxious, and I get depressed about it.

The real work of therapy begins here. All previous time has been spent setting the stage.

It seems incongruous that Centrum would not be aware, yet it is not uncommon for this to be the case.

Centrum, are you now aware of your conscious concern? YES Centrum, are you willing to cooperate, to do some work as I guide you and teach you how, with the objective of your having normal tearing in your eyes? YES Centrum, do you have the ability to look at memories of past experiences? I THINK SO Centrum, do you have the ability to communicate with other parts of your mind? YES Then, Centrum, please use those abilities, and any other ability you may have, to investigate this problem of dry eyes. Find out when the problem began and why it began. The objective at this point is for you, Centrum, to understand the beginning and continuation of this problem. Centrum, is my request clear to you? YES Then Centrum, please accomplish that task to the limit of your ability and let me know by writing the word "complete" on the chalkboard when you have done so. COMPLETE Centrum, do you believe you now understand the cause of this dry eye problem? YES

Centrum, is some part or parts of your mind causing your eyes to be dry? NO Centrum, is this problem a consequence of some experience you had? YES Centrum, did you 'learn' to experience dry eyes, as opposed to it being caused by physical injury? NO ... YES ... MAYBE

Note that the causal 'experience' could have been a physical accident. Centrum is very literal in responding.

Centrum, our bodies contain three classes of muscles. Skeletal muscles are those muscles we can control consciously, for example to lift a finger. Smooth muscles are those muscles that regulate the process of digestion and the other vital functions. Smooth muscles control the pattern of blood flow in the body and have a lot to do with respiration. In fact, the glands themselves are made up of smooth muscle. The third class muscles, cardiac muscles, are those muscles in the heart that pump blood to the extremities. We do not have conscious control of either smooth muscles or cardiac muscles. Centrum, in some manner the glands responsible for the creation of tears in your eyes are not functioning properly. We know they

A typical narration I use to introduce the concept of smooth muscle action.

are capable of functioning properly because they respond to medication. Please investigate this situation, Centrum. See if you can find out what is going on. Communicate with other parts of your mind that are involved in any way, review associated memories, and do anything else you know to do to get to the root of this problem. Centrum, is my request clear to you? YES Please let me know when you have completed the task by the word "complete" on the chalkboard. COMPLETE

Centrum, do you believe you now understand the actual cause of this problem? I DON'T KNOW Centrum, do you believe the problem is due to some unconscious control issue? NO

Centrum, please investigate the possibility that some part of your mind is actively interfering with the tearing for some reason. Is my request clear to you? YES Centrum, let me know when you have completed the task. COMPLETE Centrum, is some part of your mind interfering with the tearing process or preventing tearing from occurring? YES Centrum, are you in communication with that part? I THINK SO Then Centrum, please communicate with that part in this way: First, listen to the part. Learn what you need to know to be able to take the second step, which will be to educate the part about present life conditions. Centrum, that part is stuck back there in time, using its influence in your best interest as it understands your best interest. By listening, you can learn what you need to know to be able to educate that part about present life conditions and needs. Centrum, is that request clear to you? YES Please let me know when you have completed the communication. COMPLETE Centrum, were you successful in that task? I THINK SO ... I HOPE SO

Centrum, is that part now willing for you to have normal tearing? THEY WANT TO BE

Centrum, would it be okay for you to know consciously about the work you have been doing – for you to have the associated memories and the understanding of the way those memories have affected your life? OKAY Then, Centrum, please elevate that information to consciousness now and let me know by the word "complete" when you have done so. COMPLETE

Lorrie, does all of that make sense to you? *I think so.* Lorrie, please rouse yourself from trance and share with me, if you are willing to do so, what you just learned.

I learned that Centrum was pleading with them to perform. It made me tear a little bit.

THIRD SESSION

Centrum, are you willing to continue this work with the objective of eliminating the dry eye problem? YES Then, Centrum, please reinvestigate this problem. Set the stage for us to continue by pulling together all of the known information. Let me know when you have done so by the word "complete" on the chalkboard. COMPLETE Identify any part of your mind that might still be interfering with the normal tearing process. COMPLETE Centrum, did you identify any part or parts? I THINK SO ... FOUR

Centrum, are you in communication with all four of those parts? YES Centrum, please select one of those four parts and proceed in this way: First, Centrum, listen to the part. Learn what you need to know to be able to educate the part about present life circumstances. Let me know by the word "complete" when you have accomplished this task. COMPLETE Centrum, were you successful in that task? I THINK SO

It's as though "they" are alter personalities. A concept that frequently occurs to me. Also notice that Centrum responded in the plural, when my guidance of the process had only focused on one part.

I have elected to repeat these instructions, even though it might not have been necessary. I was acting on instinct, which I have found advisable to do in many situations.

Centrum, please select a second part and repeat the same process. COMPLETE Centrum, were you successful in persuading that part to meet present life needs? I DON'T KNOW Centrum, please communicate further with that part. Be sure you understand where that part is coming from, what it believes and why it believes what it believes. Then, please communicate to that part full understanding of your present life situation and the negative consequence of the influence that part has been exerting. COMPLETE Centrum, were you successful this time? I THINK SO Centrum, please repeat the same sequence with the third part and let me know when you have done so. COMPLETE Centrum, were you successful with this part? YES

If you think of Centrum as another person, with limited knowledge and skills – and Centrum does have limited knowledge and skills – you will find things flow smoother.

Centrum, please repeat the sequence again with the fourth part. COMPLETE Were you successful with that fourth part? I THINK SO

Centrum, it is often true that when one part has been identified and resolved, it then, and only then, becomes possible to identify some other part. Please search, Centrum; identify any remaining part, or parts, that have in the past, or might in the future, cause this tearing problem to continue. COMPLETE Did you identify any remaining part or parts? YES, A LOT Centrum, are you in communication with all the parts? (No response)

Centrum, I ask that you repeat that same process of listening and educating with each of those remaining parts of your mind. Work with each part, in turn, one at a time, and let me know when you have completed that task. COMPLETE Centrum, were you successful in persuading all of those parts to your way of thinking? YES Centrum how many parts, did you identify and communicate with? A LOT

Perhaps I did not wait long enough for a response. I assumed Centrum was in communication with the parts because of past performance. As it turned out, my assumption was correct.

Identifying and resolving one part can make it possible to identify another part that was not known before. Please search once again to identify any remaining part. COMPLETE Did you identify one or more such parts? YES ... ONE Centrum, do you know what to do? YES Centrum, please accomplish that task and let me know by the word "complete" when you have done so. COMPLETE Centrum, were you successful? YES

Would it be okay for you to have full conscious awareness and understanding of the work you just did? SURE Then, Centrum, please elevate that awareness to consciousness.

Lorrie, does it make sense to you? *I think so. Some of it was random and ridiculous.*

Centrum, has the tearing problem now been resolved? GOD ... I HOPE SO Centrum, as a test, communicate with all of those involved parts of your mind and bring on some tears right now. *I feel some tearing. Not a lot, a little bit.*

Centrum, as a test of this work, permit and/or cause tears as though you were crying. *It's been so long since I cried.*

Centrum, are you now free to cry? YES Is there any remaining barrier to your crying? NO Lorrie, do you believe that is true? *Yes, I do. It's so painful, I try not to cry.* Are there now adequate tears for lubrication? *Yes.*

Centrum, do you believe you will tear normally the next time you cry? YES

Centrum, please communicate to consciousness the basis for your belief that you will tear normally. OKAY ... COMPLETE

Lorrie, what do you believe now? Do you believe you will tear normally the next time you cry?

Something has happened in my head today. My subconscious has had a message. I now understand that it is necessary that I have had this problem. In a sense, it made sense then. It was talking to the parts and not accepting excuses.

Centrum, do you now believe all parts of your mind engage in normal functioning? THE BEST I CAN Centrum, is there more to be accomplished to achieve what you consciously want regarding this eye tearing problem? MAYBE

Centrum, I ask that you continue the work between now and the next time we meet. Are you willing to do so? YES

Martha – A Case of Unrelenting, Minimally Productive Coughing

Martha was a 51-year-old female suffering from minimally productive, yet persistent coughing, occurring in spells of one-to-three minutes, on about ten-minute intervals during the previous six weeks. A medical workup was negative except to reveal that the cough was a means of eliminating mucus. The evaluating physician also mentioned asthma without explanation. Martha was in a stable marriage with two grown children, both of whom were sources of stress in her life. Stress also derived from situations that were compounded by financial considerations. This patient had been seen previously for other problems and was therefore familiar with the concepts and procedures of Subliminal Therapy. She required no introduction or review.

FIRST SESSION

Centrum, are you aware of your conscious concern about the coughing and how it is disrupting your life? YES Centrum, are you willing to cooperate in this work with the objective of eliminating that cough? YES

Then Centrum, please conduct that investigation as you have done previously, and also, consider the possibility that the action of smooth muscle is occluding airways in ways that might prompt unnecessary coughing. Please identify those parts of your mind that are causing the coughing to occur. COMPLETE Centrum, did you identify one or more parts of your mind? YES How many parts did you identify? TWO

Centrum, do you believe you now understand why those parts are causing this recurring cough to happen? YES

More traditional therapies would likely pause at this point to inquire about the reasons just exposed. Since I have no need to know at this juncture, I accept the word of Centrum and proceed.

Please Centrum, select one of those two parts and communicate with that part as you have done on previous occasions. First, listen, and then educate that part about present reality. Let me know when you have completed the task. COMPLETE Centrum, were you successful? YES

Centrum, pleases repeat the process with the second of the two parts. Let me know when you have completed the task. COMPLETE Were you successful in this case also? YES Centrum, let there be full conscious understanding and awareness of the work you have just completed. COMPLETE

Martha, are you satisfied with your understanding of the work Centrum has just done?

Although, as the therapist, I have no need to know, it seems consistently advisable to engineer awareness on the part of the patient.

The coughing is to clear out mucus from my lungs. It does not have anything to do with asthma.

Centrum, is that correct? YES Centrum, the creation of mucus is mediated by smooth muscle acting through the glands of the body. Centrum, I ask that you investigate the possibility of intervening in some way that will block, or stop the process of that generation. COMPLETE STRESS

I deviated from normal protocol at this point, as I often do with patients who are proficient with ST.

Centrum, how old were you when the process of mucus generation began? 23 IN COLLEGE VERY STRESSFUL EXPERIENCE LED TO PRODUCTIVE COUGH

Unexpected, unrequested and welcome insight provided by Centrum.

Centrum, is the present situation a replication of the 23-year-old experience? YES

Centrum, please identify the part, or parts, that are responsible for the generation of mucus in response to stress. ONE Centrum, do you know what to do? YES Then Centrum, please accomplish that task. COMPLETE. Centrum, were you successful? YES Centrum, please elevate understanding of that work to consciousness. COMPLETE

SECOND SESSION – Two days later

Martha reported, *There has been a marked reduction in both the frequency of the episodes and the intensity, yet the coughing has continued.*

Centrum, are you aware the coughing has continued? YES Centrum, please investigate to determine why it has continued. COMPLETE Centrum, did you identify one or more parts of your mind that have continued to actively cause coughing? YES How many? ONE Centrum, do you know what to do? YES Then, Centrum, please do the work you know to do to eliminate that influence. COMPLETE Centrum, were you successful? YES

In a telephone conversation on the following day, Martha reported almost complete remission of the coughing.

Fred – Compromised Sexual Relations in Consequence of Early Molestation

Fred was a 37-year-old male who wanted normal sexual relationships with women and, ideally, a committed long-term relationship, but found himself embittered toward women. *"For me, sex is pure animal sex; there's no emotion."* He reported a problematic relationship with his mother since he could remember, but was not able to account for its being problematic. His relationships with women were complicated by a compulsion to investigate their history, to find out all about them in order to identify their faults. Almost as an aside, he mentioned having a small penis and wondered if that had anything to do with his difficulty. At the time of the following excerpt, Fred had addressed three other issues; he and Centrum were well-acquainted with the process of ST.

This excerpt illustrates the way Centrum can be engaged to uncover information that is deeply buried in the unconscious domain.

SEVENTH SESSION

I don't feel shame about my penis size when I'm with a girl; I function very well. If I could choose, I'd have a larger one, but that's the way it is. Yet, I believe it has some influence on my behavior. And too, something happened when I was about 4 or 5 years old.

Centrum, have you been listening? YES Centrum, do you believe that the 4-year-old experience you mentioned was pivotal in leading you to stray from reality in your thinking about women? YES Centrum, I believe it is in your best interest to uncover that experience because only then can the influence be resolved. I am aware that you, or some part of your mind, are strongly protective in denying the conscious memory, because you have no memory of the event.

Two possible avenues of inquiry were apparent. My choice of the 4-year-old experience was instinctual; I cannot logically justify the selection.

And so, I wonder if it is possible for you, Centrum, to communicate with me about this without conscious awareness of what is communicated. Centrum, do you believe that is possible? YES

I also deviated from the usual protocol without conscious consideration of why.

Centrum, do you know how to make that happen? YES Centrum, are you willing to do so, are you willing to work with me without conscious awareness? YES Are you consciously willing for that to happen? *Yes.*

Although I opted to seek information without conscious awareness of content, I have not ever been successful in obtaining information in that way.

Centrum, do you have a memory of what happened when you were about 4 years old? YES Centrum, are you willing to tell me, are you willing for me to know? YES Centrum, does any part of your mind object to that happening? YES

Then Centrum, please communicate with that part, and persuade that part to permit the communication between you and me. This is so important to your future. OKAY Centrum, did you succeed in persuading that part? YES Centrum, please tell me what happened while your conscious mind was asleep. Is it possible for you to do that now? I AM TRYING

I got three images, one was sleeping with mother. I saw her without underwear on. I believe she was awake and showing herself. One time, I was older, I was thinking about sex, I took a shower and had an erection and I played with it. The circumcision and the infection. It was painful to urinate, and I cried.

This was not a coherent statement; however, it seemed informative to him so I went on without questioning the content.

Centrum, is there more to what happened than those three things? YES Centrum, are you able to tell me? YES Then please do so. (No response)

Centrum, would it be easier for you to write what you need to say? NO Centrum, let me have one word at a time. (No response) Centrum, are you working on the subject of communicating the information to me? YES Centrum, would it help if I asked specific questions? YES

Centrum, was there one specific event, one pivotal event, responsible for the present situation? YES Centrum did this event involve your mother? YES Centrum, was anyone else involved? Was anyone else present when that happened? (Fred turned his head slowly from left to right and back again)

Fred had mentioned circumcision and I was asking specific questions.

Centrum, was this event your circumcision? I DON'T KNOW

Centrum, was what happened sexual in any way? YES Centrum, did your mother do something sexual to you? YES Centrum, did your mother touch your genitals? YES Centrum, do you believe she did so for her own gratification? YES Centrum, please tell me some words to describe how you felt when she did that. GUILT SHAME ANGER Centrum, did you then believe it was your fault, that you were to blame? NO Centrum, did you then conclude this was the way all females are? YES Centrum, do you now, as an adult, know that is not true? NO

I really hate them! Fred, did you have conscious awareness of all things that happened in this last interaction with Centrum? *Yes.*

I should have asked if he *believed* he had awareness.

EIGHTH SESSION

Centrum, I believe it is very important for you, Centrum, to have full, clear memory of what happened with your mother. Therefore, I ask that you exert strong effort to retrieve it. Are you willing to do that? YES Then, please do so.

Note that I am not asking for conscious memory, only that Centrum have the necessary memories.

Centrum, is that memory now clear and complete? (Fred's head turned full to the left, followed by unusual side-to-side motion of his left hand resting on his thigh. Some minutes later, his head turned forty-five degrees toward the center) Centrum, are you still involved in the process I requested of you? YES Centrum, are you still making progress? YES I DON'T FIND ANYTHING

Centrum, do you still believe your mother molested you sexually? NOT SURE Centrum, do you still believe something of a sexual nature happened, not necessarily with your mother? YES

The root of the problem might well have been a dream.

Centrum, you reported that since our last session you have slept better and have had better concentration at work, and with a clearer mind. Do you believe the uncovering that you have been doing is responsible for the improvement? POSSIBLY, YES

I posed this question to set the stage for the line of questioning that follows.

Centrum, is one or more parts of your mind still blocking that important memory from consciousness? YES How many parts are involved? ONE Centrum, are you able to communicate with that part? NO Are you willing to communicate with that part? YES Centrum, is the part willing to communicate with you? NO Centrum, is that part willing to receive information from you without the requirement for personal exposure? YES Then Centrum, please communicate information *to* that part about current problems in your life that may be resolved by the evaluation of this experience in the light of mature knowledge and understanding. Centrum, is that part now willing to communicate with *you*? YES Then Centrum, please persuade the part to permit this memory, so that we can heal the wound.

This sequence of questions has proved highly effective in engineering communications between Centrum and an uncooperative part.

Two things came to my mind:

1. At 5 years old, when I was taking a shower, I was playing with my penis. It was hard, and my mother came in. I was confused whether I should show mother or not. She continued to shower me, said I should go ahead and play with it myself, and she would come back.

This is a reinterpretation of the story related above. Which is accurate? I don't know. Further work is necessary and the bottom line is that it doesn't matter. It only matters what he understood at an unconscious level.

2. I was afraid one night and I came to my mother's bedroom and the door was closed and locked. I knew something was happening inside, and I cried. That was when I was 3 or 4 years old.

Georgia – A Case of Guilt for Having Been Born

Georgia was a 30-year-old female who presented with multiple issues. Her primary concern in this, her fifth session, was an underlying sense of guilt that had pervaded her life since she could remember, and which had become intolerable in recent weeks following a disagreement with her mother. She described this sense of guilt as being related to having been born because of awareness of the problems her birth created for her mother. This excerpt is presented in illustration of the fallibility of Centrum, and of the manner in which Centrum can be persuaded to reframe and re-evaluate, just as it's possible with others.

SESSION FIVE

Centrum, are you aware of the sense of guilt for having been born that you have been consciously expressing? YES Centrum, do you agree with your conscious opinion that such guilt is dysfunctional, misplaced, unnecessary, and really doesn't make sense now? NO

Centrum, do you believe that guilt serves some useful purpose in your life? YES Centrum, would it be okay for you to know, consciously, what that purpose is? NO

Centrum, how old were you when you were first aware of the feelings of guilt? 6, 4, 12

Centrum, did something happen when you were 6 years old, 4 years old and 12 years old? YES Centrum, I believe it is in your best interest to have conscious awareness of those events, for you to consciously remember the events. Are you willing for that to happen? NO

Since Georgia was experienced with ST, I thought preparatory steps might be unnecessary, and I bypassed them with unfortunate consequences.

133

Centrum, I believe it is in your best interest to understand the cause of problems, so that you can evaluate those causes in the light of mature understanding, especially if the causing event originated in childhood. Do you agree with me? YES Centrum, do you agree that the guilt is an example of such an issue? YES

By leading Centrum down a logical path to a conclusion in accord with mine, my lead forced Centrum to consider the issue in a different light. Or did I?

Centrum, did you reconsider your position regarding the value of that guilt in your life? NO Centrum, until this point, you have been – as I observe things – rational and mature in your thinking. I don't understand how you are thinking about the guilt. Are you willing to help me understand? YES

It would seem I did not. Centrum still holds the same opinion.

Centrum, guilt can serve useful purpose if it is based on a mistake that was made and there is need to be reminded to avoid repeating that mistake. Do you agree with me? YES

Centrum, did you have choice about being born? YES

Wow! Now there is a challenge …

Centrum, was it possible for you to have avoided being born? YES … NO Centrum, how could you have avoided being born? DEATH

Well, at least Centrum is being logical in an absolute sense.

Centrum, does your life have meaning today? YES Centrum, is it good that you have lived? YES

I decided to enter through another door.

Centrum, please tell me what happened, and what you learned from what happened, when you were 4 years old. Help me to understand. PAIN Centrum, please elaborate. You can speak to me. Please tell me. I DON'T KNOW JUST PAIN

Notice that in response to my request, Centrum has become more verbose in responding.

Centrum, was it physical pain? NO EMOTIONAL. IT WAS A SINFUL RELATIONSHIP. FATHER WAS MARRIED TO ANOTHER WOMAN

Centrum says there is another thing. When it became known that my parents weren't married we had to change school. The other kids would not speak to me.

Centrum, what did that mean to you then? What did it say about you? THAT I WAS BETTER OFF ALONE

Centrum, what happened when you were 6 years old? THEY SPIT ON MY LUNCH Centrum, what did that mean to you then, when you were 6 years old? PAIN Centrum, what message was being communicated by the kids? I WAS UNWANTED

Centrum, what happened when you were 12 years old? HAIR Centrum, please explain what you mean, tell me what happened. I HAD FACIAL PROBLEMS, ACNE AND HAIR Centrum, how did those experiences relate to your being born ? UNWANTED

Georgia, stay in trance and reflect on this question: Who wanted you when you were born?

I guess no one … No, my mother says she did. I caused a lot of problems. You know, that's absurd!

Centrum, do you agree that it is absurd? NO Georgia, it is not unusual for pregnancies to occur in situations that create problems for the parents. However, once the child is born, even the unwanted children are usually welcomed and loved.

Notice the change in her conscious thinking. Now that change must be incorporated in the unconscious domain.

If I hadn't been born, mother would not have gotten into such a long relationship with a jerk (my father). I had to change schools when it was learned that mother was not married to my father. I feel guilty, even today, when I tell someone about going on vacation, or when I buy things for myself, or when I'm not working twelve hours a day.

All this did not make logical sense to me; however, it did to her and that was all that mattered.

Centrum, do you believe these burdens all tie back to the guilt for being born? YES Centrum, is that fair? NO

Centrum's first about-face.

Centrum, did you have the option, the choice, to not live? NO

Centrum's second change of mind.

Centrum, we can *feel* responsible without *being* responsible. In fact, we can only *be* responsible if we are in control. Do you agree with that statement? YES

Again, I am leading Centrum to a logical conclusion.

Centrum, were you, in fact, in control about your birth? NO Centrum, do you agree that you were not responsible for your birth? YES Centrum, do you now agree the guilt you have been feeling is not based in reality? YES Centrum, does any part of your mind still believe you were guilty for having been born? YES ... NO Centrum, how many parts of your mind still believe that somehow you were guilty for having been born? NONE Centrum, what was the "yes" part of your previous answer? FREE Centrum, are you now free of that guilt? YES

The final capitulation. The only step required now is to ensure that all parts of her mind agree with Centrum.

Tim – A Case of Panic Attacks Leading to Agoraphobia

Tim was a 72-year-old man who presented with agoraphobia in consequence of panic attacks that began at about the age of 7 years. He had undergone *"every treatment I ever heard of, including forty years of Freudian psychotherapy,"* in attempts to rid himself of the panic attacks, which were disabling in multiple aspects of his life. In his way of thinking, Tom equated his panic attacks with agoraphobia and he expressed them interchangeably.

SESSION 2

Centrum, do you agree the panic attacks should be addressed at this time? YES Centrum, are you willing to communicate with me via the chalkboard? *It's like a shadow.* Centrum, is some part resisting this work? YES Centrum, are you in communication with that part? YES Centrum, do you believe we should pursue the elimination of panic attacks? YES

Centrum, please communicate with the resisting part. Persuade that part to permit the work to go forward.

Is my request clear to you? YES Then Centrum, please complete that task to the limit of your ability and let me know by the word "complete" when you have done so. COMPLETE Centrum, were you successful? YES

Centrum, please investigate the origin of the panic attacks, doing so with or without conscious awareness. One or more parts of your mind were created in that situation in which the panic attacks originated. Learn whatever you need to know about that experience. COMPLETE Centrum, do you believe you now understand the origin of the panic attacks? NO

Centrum, how old were you when the panic attacks began? SEVEN Centrum, please identify the part or parts of your mind that were formed when you were 7 years old and that have continued to cause the panic attacks. Is that request clear to you? YES Then Centrum, please identify those parts. COMPLETE Centrum, did you identify one or more such parts? YES How many did you identify? THREE And Centrum, are you in communication with all three of the parts? YES Centrum, please select one of those three parts and communicate with that part in this special way. First listen. Learn what you need to know to be able to educate that part about present reality. When you know what you need to know please accomplish that educational process. Let that part understand the negative consequences of its influence. Grow that part up and persuade it to your way of thinking. Is my request clear? YES Then let me know when you have completed the task. COMPLETE Centrum, were you successful in that task? YES NO

> By asking Centrum to tell me his age at the onset of the panic attacks, I was forcing Centrum to focus on a single event from which further inquiry could develop.

Centrum, does that part believe the panic attacks serve useful purpose in your life? YES Centrum, do you agree? NO Then Centrum, please engage the part further. Learn why the part believes what it believes, and based on that understanding, persuade the part to your way of thinking. COMPLETE Were you successful? YES

> Avoid assuming Centrum holds a given opinion; be sure. Ask.

Centrum, would it be okay for you to understand, at a conscious level of awareness, the work you just accomplished? YES Then Centrum, please elevate that understanding to consciousness now. LOST Centrum, this is a yes or no question. Do you now have full conscious understanding? NO Centrum, it seems advantageous, but not essential, for there to be conscious awareness and understanding of the work that is completed. Do you believe it is in your best interest to have that knowledge, that memory and understanding, consciously? YES Centrum, is some part of your mind resisting that conscious awareness, perhaps to protect you in some way? YES Are you in communication with that part? YES Then Centrum, persuade that part to permit conscious awareness and understanding and let me know when you have done so by the word "complete". COMPLETE Were you successful in persuading that part? YES Centrum, let that understanding become conscious now.

A little boy is going to be run over by horses.

Centrum, was that the event responsible for the panic attacks? YES Centrum, was that little boy you? YES Centrum, it is certainly understandable that your reaction in that situation was to experience panic. That experience of panic seemingly became associated with some cue and you have since continued to respond with panic in reaction to that stimulus. Centrum, does this make sense to you? YES Centrum, do you agree that that reaction of panic is inappropriate in your life now as an adult? YES

The words were fuzzy, like in a cloud. I wanted a clear picture of the words.

SESSION 3

During the past week I have not had any panic attacks and I have felt less anxious as well. In the past I have had panic attacks on Highway 15 at a particular place. I

have had to pull over and then go back. If I go forward the panic attacks increase in intensity. I have not yet tested Highway 15.

Centrum, are you willing to continue this work with the objective of completely eliminating the panic attacks? YES Centrum, you have expressed conscious concern about the fuzzy answers. Please investigate those answers and if possible make them clear and sharp. FEAR Centrum, what is feared? DEATH Centrum, does some part of your mind fear this work might cause death? YES Centrum, do you fear this work might cause death? NO Centrum, are you in communication with that part of your mind that does fear? I DON'T KNOW Centrum, is that part willing to communicate with you? YES

I might have ignored Tim's statement of concern about the image being unclear. I might instead have guided Centrum to the next step of the usual sequence. I hung in there because I sensed his conscious preoccupation with it would interfere with the ST process.

All kinds of squirreling things are going on.

Centrum, please listen to that part that fears death. When you understand more precisely what the part fears, and why it fears what it fears, reassure the part so that it is no longer afraid. Educate the part about present reality. COMPLETE Centrum, is that part still afraid? NO Tim, is the chalkboard clear now? *No.*

Note that I progressively rely on Centrum to accomplish specific steps without taking the time to cover each step.

Centrum, please find out what is going on. Perhaps there is another part of your mind interfering with this work. Do all that you know to do to correct the situation.

And in each case something came up. Something happened to my body and I had to go to the hospital.

My inner bulldog has come out and is determined to resolve the clarity issue. Problem is, I don't know what to do, so I turn it over to Centrum in a general sense.

Centrum, it will be necessary to identify every part of your mind that is interfering. Please do so now. COMPLETE Did you identify any remaining parts? YES, TWO Centrum, are you in communication with both parts? NO Are you in communication with either part? YES Then Centrum, please communicate with that part in the same manner as before, first listen, then educate. COMPLETE Were you successful in persuading that part to your way of thinking? YES Centrum, is the second part now willing to communicate with you? YES Then Centrum, please repeat that same protocol and let me know when you have done so. COMPLETE Were you successful with the second part? YES Tim, is the chalkboard now clear? *No.*

Centrum, are you aware of the interfering influence? YES Centrum, please find out what the source is, then eliminate that influence by communicating with the responsible part. Is my request clear to you? YES Then please accomplish that task to the limit of your ability. COMPLETE Centrum, were you successful? YES Tim, is the chalkboard now clear? *It's a little clearer.*

Centrum, are you willing to continue this work to accomplish clear communications? YES Centrum, do you know what to do to achieve clear communications via the chalkboard? NO *I touched the chalkboard and got shocked.*

SESSION 4

I went to that place on Highway 15 and the panic attacks returned. The fear of dying came up like gangbusters. I didn't know if I would survive it. I exited the first ramp and went to Wal-Mart for ice cream as a way to calm down a little. The beginning of a panic attack occurred while I was driving later on in the day. A part of me does not know this treatment will not kill me.

The panic reaction is still there. The work is not complete. There were hints of giving up on his part, hints that were ignored by me.

Note: the rest of the session was devoted to other subject matter, following a discussion of his opening statement.

SESSION 5

Tim was very tense at the beginning of the session; he was talking in a semi-compulsive way. *I feel locked in because of the agoraphobia and I am having a problem*

140

with the wife too. I had one additional experience of the agoraphobia while driving. I asked Centrum to help me and I was able to go forward, instead of having to go back as before.

I am always pleased to learn that the patient is interacting with Centrum on their own.

Centrum, are you aware of that recent experience of agoraphobia? YES Centrum, are you willing to continue this work? YES Centrum, those experiences are the consequence of the influence of one or more parts of your mind, parts that came into existence in different experiences during the course of your life. Please identify those parts and let me know when you have done so. I DON'T KNOW

Centrum, do you agree that the panic attacks were caused by one or more parts of your mind? YES Centrum, are you capable of identifying those parts? You have been successful in the past, are you capable now? I THINK SO Then Centrum, please do all that you know to do to accomplish that goal. YES! Centrum, did you identify one or more parts? YES, FOUR Centrum, are you in communication with all four? YES Then Centrum, please select one of the four parts and repeat that protocol, listen, then educate. Ensure that part understands the negative consequences of its influence and persuade that part to support present life needs. COMPLETE Centrum, were you successful? YES

Here, I am simply rephrasing my request, hopefully to guide Centrum to approach the issue from another perspective.

Centrum, you stated when we last met, as you went out the door, that some part does not know "this therapy will not kill me." Does that part exist? YES Are you in communication with that part? YES Then Centrum, please communicate with that part, listen then educate, grow that part up. COMPLETE Were you successful? YES Centrum, does any other part of your mind fear this work will kill you? NO

I had made note of this comment, picking up on the literal use of "part" to describe his insight. I do not remember my rationale bringing it to the table at this point. Perhaps it was instinctual.

Centrum, please select a second of those original four parts and repeat the same protocol as before. REPEAT Centrum, minutes ago you identified four parts of

The "Repeat" response was unexpected. Perhaps Centrum was preoccupied with thought about the previous question.

your mind that were influencing the panic attacks to occur. You communicated with, and presumably resolved, one of the parts. I now ask that you select one of the remaining three parts and repeat the protocol. Is my request clear? YES Please let me know. OKAY Were you successful? YES Centrum, please repeat that same process with part number three of the original four. (A long delay ensued) Centrum, are you still in the process of completing that task? YES Centrum, are you having difficulty with that task? YES

Centrum, are there two remaining parts of your mind that are disposed to cause the panic attacks to continue? *"ROUG" came across the screen.*

Centrum, you say you are willing to continue this work, so let's start over. Centrum, please investigate this entire situation involving the panic attacks. Identify any part or parts of your mind that have in the past, or might in the future, cause the panic attacks to continue and let me know when you have done all that you know to do. CRAZY Centrum, did you identify one or more such parts? YES How many? ONE Centrum, do you know what to do? YES Then please do so. *Pictures on the wall are confusing, I don't know what they mean.*

At a loss to make meaning out of Centrum's response, I elected to begin again.

I chose not to be distracted by the "Crazy" response.

Centrum, do you know what to do in this situation? YES Then please do so. YES Were you successful? YES Centrum, are you willing for there to be full conscious understanding, full awareness of the memories and understanding of the effect of those memories? YES Then Centrum, please elevate that understanding to consciousness now and let me know when you have done so by the word "complete". COMPLETE Tim, did you just learn what you want to know?

It was me as a little boy. I saw an advertising board that said "you are going to die." It scared me. It stuck in my head. A girl named "Pinky" lived across the street from me. She took me to see a horror movie.

Those two events caused me to be afraid all the time. I don't know where the night stuff came from, and when I bent over to catch a ball, my heart accelerated. I had to go to the hospital where they gave me some real red stuff to slow it down.

I know now that fear accelerates heart rate. I did not know that them. I thought I was going to be dead.

Tim, does that reaction of panic make sense to you consciously? Does it have a name value in your life today? *Not much.*

It is no doubt apparent to the reader that this work is not complete. This excerpt was included here before treatment had been concluded to show an unusually complex pattern of responses and problems. In my experience, cases of this complexity are encountered in only one out of about twenty cases. I am optimistic about the outcome.

Becky – A Case of Anxiety with Occasional Panic Attacks

Becky was a 47-year-old female who presented with anxiety of childhood origin and infrequent panic attacks. Her situation was complicated by grief from the recent death of a family member, as well as by claustrophobia.

SECOND SESSION

This one-hour session was devoted to guiding Becky through the grief procedure as described in my book, *Foundations of Clinical Hypnosis* (2008). Subliminal Therapy was not employed in this session.

THIRD SESSION (Two-hour duration)

Becky reported "remarkable" relief from the burden of grief she had been carrying, feeling well prepared to move on. She had read my introductory book on Subliminal Therapy and was "enthralled" by what she learned. Communication with Centrum was easily established.

Centrum, are you aware of your conscious concern about the anxiety, and the way it interferes with your life? YES Centrum, are you willing to cooperate to do some work as I guide you and teach you how, with the objective of eliminating the anxiety? NO Centrum, do you believe the anxiety serves a useful purpose in your life? YES Centrum, would it be okay for you to have conscious knowledge of that purpose? YES Centrum, please elevate that understanding to consciousness now.

> Although not commonly true, Centrum may not be aware of the problem.

> Since Centrum is willing for there to be conscious awareness, something else is going on.

Scribbling on the chalkboard.

Centrum, is some part interfering, preventing conscious awareness? YES FEAR Centrum, are you in communication with that resisting part? NO Are you willing to communicate with that part? NO Centrum, do you fear that part? NO YES

There is a lot of door slamming.

Jack – A Case of Compulsive Behavior

Jack was a married, 58-year-old man "haunted by a sexual issue" for thirty-five years; he was compelled to look down to check that his penis was still there, a check that was required every few minutes. Jack also presented other, much less significant compulsions; however, "it" was the big one. He was a family oriented man, much embarrassed by his behavior and motivated to change it. As will become significant later, he was never in the armed services.

At age 3 to 4 years, Jack would not urinate, requiring hot baths to cause urination without his control. His father was bi-sexual, often wearing no clothes around the house, and his mother reported finding his father on top of him on one occasion. These bits of memory were most of what he initially recalled of his childhood.

Session one was an unremarkable session of history-taking and goal establishment. He stated, *"I think the purpose of the compulsions, all of them, is to make me feel ashamed, dysfunctional and anxious, and to avoid thinking about something else."*

This case is an excellent illustration of the advantages afforded when Centrum is eloquent in responses.

SECOND SESSION (Three-hour duration)

Jack had read my little book on ST and after teaching him the skill of self-hypnosis, the concepts of Subliminal Therapy were reviewed and communication with Centrum was established.

Centrum, are you aware of your conscious concerns about your compulsive behavior? NO Jack, please express aloud and in your own words why you are bothered by the compulsion to check that your penis is there. *(Narration was provided.)*

Centrum, are you now aware of your conscious concern? YES Centrum, are you willing to cooperate, to do some work as I guide you and teach you how, with the objective of eliminating that compulsive behavior? YES Centrum, are you capable of remembering events all through your life? SOME Centrum are you capable of communicating with other parts of your mind? I THINK SO

Centrum, please use whatever abilities you have to conduct an investigation into the origin of this compulsive behavior. Communicate with other parts of your mind, review memories, use whatever abilities you have to accomplish the task. Centrum, is my request clear to you? YES Then Centrum, please complete that task to the limit of your ability and let us know when you have done so by writing the word "complete" on the chalkboard. COMPLETE Centrum, do you believe you now understand the cause of that compulsive behavior? YES

Centrum, how old were you when the compulsions began? (No response) Centrum, do you know how old you were? NO Centrum, please investigate, find out how old you were. COMPLETE Centrum, how old were you? LESS THAN 1 YEAR OLD Centrum, is the problem in consequence of something that happened to you, that someone did to you? YES

Notice the literal communication. Centrum could not answer the question, so no answer was forthcoming.

Centrum, when that happened to you, a part of your mind came into existence, a part that has continued to influence your life. Perhaps it happened more than once, or related things happened, in which case other parts of your mind also were formed. Centrum, please identify those parts of your mind in preparation for communicating with them. Centrum, is my request clear to you? YES Then Centrum, please identify those parts and let me know by the word "complete" when you have done so. COMPLETE Centrum, did you identify one or more such parts? YES, THREE Centrum, are you in communication with all three of those parts? YES Centrum, please select one of the three parts and communicate with that part in this way: First listen to the part. Learn what you need to know to be able to educate that part about present reality. Centrum, that part is stuck in that time when it came into existence. It is well-intended, however, its intentions are based on its understanding of your life at that time, the understanding that was true for you when that part developed. The part is stuck in time, using its influence based on that understanding. Centrum, your task will be that of educating the part about present reality, persuading it to support the needs of your life now, as it is today.

This question about clarity is strongly advised. Were it not clear to Centrum, the process could not go forward and you might not know why.

Centrum, is that request clear to you? YES Then Centrum, please complete that communication process and let me know by the word "complete" when you have done so. STUCK

Centrum, do you believe you understand what that part believes? YES Centrum, are you still in communication with the part? YES Centrum, have you communicated the necessary information to that part? CAN'T, EVIL, CAN'T GET PAST

Centrum, Is that "evil" preventing the part from learning? PAIN, ANGER Centrum, are you experiencing pain? NO Centrum, is that first part experiencing pain? I DON'T KNOW Centrum, who is experiencing that pain? MY BODY

Centrum, please determine if an evil part is presenting part number one from learning what it needs to learn. NO SCARED PART Centrum, are you in communication with that scared part? I KNOW

Centrum, are you willing to communicate with that scared part? LET HIM, LET MY FATHER Centrum, is that evil part aware of present reality? CHILD DON'T WANT ADULT SHOULD DIE ME–HIM (FATHER) THE SAME CHILD SHOULD LIVE MUST MAKE IT COMPLETE BY DYING MYSELF BECAUSE FATHER AND I ARE THE SAME

Centrum, have those words been coming from you? YES Centrum, do you believe you should die? YES … NO

Centrum, by cooperating with me in this work, you will be resolving all of those influences from the past that are creating the current problems. It is my belief that having resolved these problems, there will no longer be any need to act compulsively. Centrum, are you willing to cooperate in this work? YES

Communication word "Stuck" was the first indication that Jack's Centrum was unusual. It provided me with information I had not asked for.

I do not understand what is going on, but I will be patient and inquire more deeply.

At this point I am suspicious that the responses are conscious responses.

Centrum, are you in communication with that part of your mind that represents evil? (No response) Centrum, I do not understand what is going on, nevertheless, I request that you communicate to that evil part of your mind information about present reality, life situation, needs, etc. COMPLETE

This was a shot in the dark, a hunch that I acted on.

Centrum, were you successful in communicating that information to that evil part? YES

Centrum, please re-engage part #1, complete the task that I requested of you minutes ago. COMPLETE Centrum, were you successful in that task? YES PAIN IS ALL I REMEMBER Centrum, did you communicate those last few words? NO

The response did not make good sense so I questioned it.

Those were my words. I was thinking them.

Centrum, do you believe you now understand what part #1 believes and why it believes what it believes? YES, RESENTMENT Centrum, is that resentment serving any useful purpose in your life? NO Centrum, does any part of your mind still believe the resentment serves useful purpose? YES Are you in communication with that part? YES Centrum, please establish communication with this part, first listen, then educate as you have been instructed before. SMALL PROBLEM, DON'T WANT ANGER, TERRIBLE, DRIVING ANGER Centrum, do you believe it is in your best interest for that anger to continue? YES

It's usually best to resolve interfering issues as they arise, then return to the basic goal.

Centrum, what is the benefit of that anger? PROTECTION KEEP HURT, PAIN, DAMAGE AWAY NO NO NO

A note of tiredness was in Centrum's communication.

Centrum do you need a break? NO

Centrum, let's proceed. Please communicate with each of those remaining two parts that we began with, one at a time, engaging them in the same way that you did the first part. With each part, first listen, then educate the part about present reality, doing so one part at a time. COMPLETE Centrum, were you successful with both of those parts in persuading them to support present life needs? NOT SURE Well Centrum, please communicate with each of those two parts to learn the answer to my question and then tell me, were you successful with both? YES Centrum, do you now have full conscious awareness of the work you've been doing, including conscious memories of the events that have been involved? YES

To be an intelligent guide of the process, I must insist on clearer answers.

Centrum, in your opinion, were you to blame for anything that happened to you as a child? YES, I WAS Centrum, I believe we can only be responsible for that which we can control. If you cannot control something, you cannot be responsible. You can, however, **feel** responsible, and I believe that's what's happening with you. Centrum, were you to blame for what happened? NO

I am pushing the process very rapidly and Centrum is still ahead of me. Centrum is doing a lot of work in the background.

Centrum, does any part of your mind still believe you were responsible? NO

Jack, if you will please rouse yourself from trance, remembering all that you choose to remember. *So tired. I feel sad.*

[A ten minute break at about the two-hour mark.]

Centrum, are you willing to continue this work? YES Centrum, the effects of events in our lives are represented by parts of our minds. Centrum, I request that you now review your life in a general way, identify those effects that are significant to your goal, and of the parts representing them, then communicate with each of those parts in the same manner as before, listening and educating, thereby reconditioning these parts to conform to the needs of your present life. Is that request clear to you, Centrum? YES Then Centrum, please communicate further to accomplish that task. COMPLETE Centrum, were you successful

At this point I decided to give Centrum greater freedom to work without my detailed knowledge or involvement.

in that task? YES Centrum, how many issues did you just resolve? I DON'T KNOW Centrum, were there a large number? YES

Centrum, please search further to identify any remaining parts that you might have missed. COMPLETE Did you identify any remaining parts, Centrum? YES, TWO Centrum, do you know what to do now? YES Then Centrum, please complete that task. COMPLETE Centrum, were you successful with both parts? YES Centrum, please repeat that same process of identifying remaining parts and resolving their unfortunate influences until none remain. COMPLETE Centrum, where you successful with all? YES

Centrum, please elevate to consciousness the memories associated with those experiences, together with understanding of how those experiences have impacted your life. (Spontaneous crying) COMPLETE Jack, did that information make sense to you? *When the final "Complete" appeared, and I cried, "He" smiled and handed the chalk to me. It was a really powerful image – like going home.*

Jack, the only actual test of this work is in the real world, of course. Yet, we can conduct a kind of test here that can be valuable. If you will, please use your imagination, now, while you are still in trance, to create situations in which, in the past, you would have experienced this resentment. *I can do them, but they fight me.*

In other words, the task of therapy is not complete.

THIRD SESSION (Two-hour duration, three days later)

Jack reported having been sick the day following the previous session. *I have been scared, but I can't clearly define why. I believe it's all about protection, protection from being penetrated, ripped open. Sometimes I will throw myself against a wall; it's like a big hand is slamming me against the wall. The movie* Sybil *tore me apart. It possibly started this.* When questioned, Jack's memory of the previous session seemed complete. He had forgotten to practice the self-hypnosis he was taught and reported he had experienced a lot of memories of his childhood. At my request, he guided himself into a trance, and responded to my suggestion for a pleasant memory, followed by a memory of mild sadness, and then spontaneously reported being in the throes of a terrible sadness.

Centrum, is it advisable to address this terrible sadness now? YES!!! TAKE MY HAND AND TAKE ME THERE

Centrum, do you know what caused that sadness to occur? YES Centrum, would it be okay for you to have conscious awareness of that cause? YES

Centrum, does any part of your mind object to you are having conscious awareness? YES Centrum, are you in communication with that resistant part? YES Centrum, do you believe it is advisable for you to have conscious awareness now? YES Then Centrum, please communicate with that resisting part. First listen. Then educate as before; persuade that part to permit this awareness. COMPLETE Centrum, were you successful? NOT SURE Centrum, please communicate further. Find out whether or not you were successful. COMPLETE Were you successful? YES Centrum, will any other part of your mind resist conscious awareness? YES How many such parts are there? I DON'T KNOW I WANT MY FATHER BACK Centrum, do you, Centrum, want your father back? YES Centrum, are you aware that that isn't possible? YES (Crying)

It's almost always advisable to check this point. Otherwise you will still get no response, but without knowing why not.

Centrum, please elevate some conscious awareness of some aspect of what happened. PAIN IN MY BACK, DOWN THERE IN MY BACK Centrum, did some man rape you? YES Centrum, was it a grown man? YES Centrum, how old was this man? I DON'T KNOW Centrum, were you a small child? YES Centrum, was the man someone you knew? *It was my father,*

It had been clear for some time that he had been raped, but I had wanted him to discover it for himself if possible. I erred here, I became impatient.

I feel it. Centrum, was it your father? (No response) Centrum, are you willing to answer that question? (No response)

Jack, please rouse yourself from trance and tell me: did you get any memories of what happened? *No, just gray sky.* We have exhausted our one-hour appointment. I have the next hour available. Would you like to continue? *Yes, I would. I have always felt dirty, bad, now I know it's not so.*

Jack, was anyone at fault for what happened? *No, it was just a tragedy ... I just want everybody to heal.* Do you believe he had the choice not to do what he did? *No, I don't believe he did.* Do you now forgive him? (Nodded "Yes") Centrum, do you also forgive your father? YES Centrum, does any part of your mind not forgive him? YES ... NONE Centrum, did you just now resolve those issues? YES

> Again, inner thinking produced a different conscious conclusion as demonstrated by the change in answers from "Yes" to "None".

What do I do now? I don't know what to do. It's all I ever prepared and trained for. I spent my whole life preparing to fight the battle; I must now find another. I don't know if I can do that. It scares me. I always knew that being a soldier was not what I wanted.

Jack, do you want to know who it was? *Yes, I do.* Centrum, are you now willing to answer the question of who it was? YES *It was my father. It doesn't even matter anymore.* Centrum, do you believe it will be necessary for you to consciously remember the experience in order to be free of it? NO Jack, are you okay with not being consciously aware? *Yes.*

> Having full conscious awareness is advantageous in several regards, but it is not always essential.

Centrum, do you know what should be done now? YES Centrum, please elevate that to consciousness. THERE'S A LOT OF POWER THERE. I MUST RELEASE IT SLOWLY Centrum, please identify any part of your mind that might resist the work you need to do. Did you identify any part or parts? YES, ONE Centrum, do you know what to do? YES Please do

> I am asking Centrum for guidance, yet I must stay involved. Experience tells me the incentive to continue the work will fade without me. Centrum seems not to like homework.

152

so. COMPLETE Centrum, were you successful? YES Centrum, please search to identify any remaining part of your mind that might resist. ONE Centrum, please handle that situation. COMPLETE Successful? YES

Centrum, please search yet again. THAT'S ALL THERE IS

At this point, I delivered a mini-lecture on the concept of this being the beginning of a new life for him. I asked what his strengths were and he responded, *People can talk to me. I can write, I'm intelligent, I have empathy, I care, and my values are clearly defined. This feels really weird, I don't know who I am right now. The toughest thing is to let go. Now it's not all or nothing. Forcing change on someone is immoral. I just couldn't function the way I was, fighting too many wars. The wars are not there anymore. The big question for me is whether the OCD will continue.*

SESSION FOUR (One-hour duration, twelve days later)

The OCD is better, but not gone. I have to believe there is a biochemical element involved. However, I'm open to the possibility there is not. The sadness is better, at least 60–70 percent better. To me, the sadness says, "I want to go home."

Centrum, are you aware of your current condition regarding the OCD and the sadness? YES Centrum, are you willing to continue this work to eliminate both? YES Centrum, please identify the specific experience or experiences in which you learned that your penis might not be there anymore. Centrum, did you succeed? NO Centrum, how old were you when you learned that lesson? VERY YOUNG ... 3 Centrum, do you now have this memory? NO ... FEELING Centrum, are you capable of finding that memory or of identifying that part of your mind? NO *In high school, when I started to ... The 'other me' is hiding.*

At this point I delivered a mini-lecture on the subject of disassociation. Centrum, please establish communication with that 'other you'. COMPLETE Centrum, please communicate with the 'other you' in a supportive way. IT WANTS TO DIE. IT DOESN'T WANT TO GO BACK. WE SHOULD LET HIM DIE, TO GO HOME. Centrum, is the 'other you' willing to listen to me? IT DOESN'T WANT TO COME BACK. Centrum, does that part have a name? JUST 'THE UNDER' OR 'THE OTHER'. WE NEED TO HIDE HIM. THEY MUSTN'T FIND HIM. THEY COME TO KILL AND BURN AND THEN LEAVE. Who is "they?" ALL MEN DESTROY. IT'S WHAT WE DO. WE MUST HANDLE HIM. IT'S WHAT WE DO. You are a man and you do not do that. I WANT TO. IT'S ALL I LIVE FOR – TO KILL AND TO FIGHT. ONLY FIGHTING IS REAL. HE DOESN'T KNOW THAT YET, TOO YOUNG TO KNOW NOW. Tell me, Centrum, doesn't pleasure also exist? NO, SMALL TIMES OF NOT FIGHTING EXIST. YOU CAN'T TRUST THE QUIET … EVER. THERE IS NO SAFETY Centrum, where and how and when did you learn that you have to fight? EVERYWHERE – ALL THE TIME. MOSTLY LATE AT NIGHT, WHEN THE WIND BLOWS IN THE TREES. THAT'S THE MOST DANGEROUS TIME, THAT'S WHEN YOU GET TORN AND DESTROYED

This was the first indication of disassociation being involved. It was not surprising, it was even to be expected.

Another hunch acted upon, and I am unable to articulate whence it came.

Still another hunch, this time, a good one.

Centrum, does love exist? (Long pause) YES, IN SOME PLACES AND REALITIES Centrum, is love worth living for? LOVE IS FRIGHTENING. I DON'T UNDERSTAND IT. IT'S MORE POWERFUL THAN ANYTHING. LOVE AND PAIN ARE TWINS, YOU CAN'T HAVE ONE WITHOUT THE OTHER. I WANT THE LITTLE BOY TO COME OUT OF THE CLOSET. I WANT TO TELL HIM SOMETHING Centrum, he can hear you. YES, LOVE IS THE MOST POWERFUL FORCE IN THE UNIVERSE. YOU MUST NOT RUN FROM IT, DESPITE THE PAIN. YOU MUST NOT RUN FROM IT, IT'S WHAT MAKES THINGS MATTER. HE MUST NOT SPEND HIS LIFE SEARCHING FOR IT.

Are you Centrum? I AM WHAT I AM, I'M ME. Do you have a name? I DON'T KNOW Would 'Protector' be a good name? NO, I AM THE ONE WHO COMES BACK TO PICK UP THE PIECES, TO SEE IF ANYTHING IS LEFT … TO TELL THEM WE CAN'T DO THIS AGAIN. I DON'T KNOW ANYTHING BUT KILLING IN MY HEAD. ALL THAT FEELS RIGHT ARE WEAPONS. I'M SO MUCH THIS ONE THING. MAYBE YOU CAN TEACH ME SOMETHING ELSE Yes! I certainly can! And I will if you will let me.

Centrum, how old was Jack when you came into existence? 3 OR 4, MAYBE Did you come into existence to fight your father? YES, HE IS NOT THE ENEMY. WHAT MADE HIM THAT WAY IS THE ENEMY OKAY. I DO CARE ABOUT PEOPLE, YOU KNOW … I CAN BRING BACK THE THINGS THAT ARE LOVE I believe you can change the effect of things that happen, even though you cannot change what happened. Do you agree with that? 'THE OTHER' WANTS TO WAIT. HE'S NOT SURE

At this point, I pointed out at some length that we are all conditioned by experience in life. I pointed out that his father had been conditioned by his life experiences, probably influenced greatly by his father, and that this is the way it happens.

I'm ready to stop for today, now. I'm so old to change, to start over. Seems really hard. I suggested he can learn new things, and that learning is not necessarily harder, it can be fun. I suggested everyone was conditioned, and that conditioning can change if we know how. I suggested he can learn how, that he is smart. After all, I pointed out, you learned the first time around, you can relearn now. I suggested that hope also exists, and pointed out that he has already begun to change. Do you recognize that? *Yes.*

I requested that Jack rouse himself from trance and pointed out, "I get confused about who is talking to me there sometimes." *Me too. I never liked to hurt anyone, not ever. It's weird, I always wanted to fight, yet realized the enemy was not any other person.*

Dean – Variations in Responses From Centrum – A

Dean was a 32-year-old man who was having severe difficulty coping with society. One might say he was odd in behavior and defiant in defending his oddness. On top of this, he obsessively masturbated and was addicted to pornography. This excerpt is from the tenth session in which he continued to address the social stress, and his life's conditioning that set him up to be defeated. It is offered here to illustrate the wide variety of responses that can occasionally be expected from Centrum.

Centrum, are you willing to continue this work to resolve the social stress problem? YES

Centrum, you consciously speak in competent terms about yourself, recognizing that there is actually, truly nothing wrong with you. Yet, when you sense rejection, you assume there is something wrong with you. Centrum, are you aware of that happening? NO
Centrum, now that I've put the matter on the table, do you agree that is happening? YES

Centrum, please identify those parts of your mind that are responsible. Identify those parts that still believe something is wrong with you, or that even question it. (No response)

Centrum, are you willing to continue this work? YES
Centrum, is some part of your mind interfering? NO

Centrum is writing in cursive. I can't read it.

Centrum, is there a reason you were writing in cursive? SCHOOL

In elementary school, I thought something was wrong with me. Centrum is telling me that is why I react so strongly when people try to control me.

At this point, I am confused and uncertain about what to do. Instinct is my only guide.

At last, a definitive answer.

The patient seems to understand, and that's what matters. I'm just floundering.

Centrum, please review the memories of those experiences in elementary school and identify those parts of your mind that were created during those experiences. COMPLETE Centrum, did you identify those parts? *Centrum says that I should trust myself.*

In the end, Centrum was correct. Rather than continue through the protocol of ST, I elected to follow Centrum's guide with the desired results being obtained. Dean is much happier now.

Penny – Variations in Responses From Centrum – B

This segment of a case was included to illustrate the flexibility in responses Centrum can present. Penny, a 56-year-old female, presented with compromised health, manifesting in frequent gastro-intestinal problems of various sorts. This segment was excerpted from the fifth treatment session.

Penny had learned in the previous session that the underlying reason for her being sick was to avoid school, a lesson she had learned from her mother at age 6. She was a school teacher at the time of treatment and had not been sick during the week following the previous treatment session. I decided to ensure completeness of the work.

I have not been sick. I think the biggest reason to be sick was to avoid the school situation.

Centrum, please search once again to identify any remaining parts of your mind that might cause you to be sick. COMPLETE Centrum, did you identify one or more such parts? YES, THREE

Centrum, have you been proactive in causing the sick-ness? THAT'S A GOOD QUESTION. EMBARRASSED TO ANSWER IT. YES

Centrum, do you mean that you have actively contri-buted to the sickness? YES, WHY NOT? IT WORKED

Centrum, do you now know why not? BEGINNING TO REALLY MIXED UP DIDN'T KNOW

Centrum, are you in communication with the three parts you identified? JUST ONE Centrum, please communicate with that part in the usual manner. First listen, then educate. Is my request clear to you? YES Then Centrum, please complete that task and let me know by the word "complete" when you have done so. COMPLETE Centrum, were you successful in that task? YES

Centrum, are you now in communication with either of the other two parts? MAYBE Centrum, I do not understand. Are you in communication with either of the parts? YES, BOTH. ONE AT A TIME

Then, Centrum, please communicate with each of them, one at a time, repeating the usual protocol that you have learned. COMPLETE Centrum, were you successful in persuading both parts to your way of thinking? YES

Centrum, please search to identify any remaining part of your mind that has or might cause you to be sick. Did you identify any such part? SEEMS LIKE NO PARTS

Centrum, do you now know why not? YES

Centrum, would it now be okay for you to understand that work at a conscious level. What you now under-stand? MAYBE NOT

Here is the first expanded response. Although I questioned its source, my instinct prevailed and I continued assuming it was valid.

Again, I questioned the source of the response, but continued based on instinct.

Centrum, does one or more parts of your mind object to your knowing consciously? *It's really not that. Centrum realizes the impact of all these years, so Centrum doesn't now have the judgment necessary to reframe the unconscious awareness. Centrum has concluded Centrum has very poor judgment and should not be allowed to make that decision.*

This response indicates that she is consciously aware of the work, but perhaps not fully so.

It also indicates an unusual self-awareness on the part of Centrum.

Centrum, people make mistakes, and you too are permitted mistakes. Hopefully, we learn from our mistakes and I believe you have learned from yours. Therefore, I repeat my question: Would it be okay for you to now have full and complete conscious aware-ness of the work you have been doing? YES Centrum, does any part of your mind object? NO Then please elevate that understanding to consciousness, includ-ing the memories of events involved and understand-ing of the continued effect of those events on your life. Let me know when you have done that by the word "complete". COMPLETE

In the first memory, I see a rack of clothing and a hand pulling them aside, revealing me hiding from school. In the second memory, I see my mother sick (and she always was). My father wanted her to go some place with him, and she used that sickness as a strategy to avoid going with him. The third memory was when I was 12 years old. I had many strep throats then. I was in private school, Catholic, strict. I was inspected every day for uniform and cleanliness, I was scrutinized and resented it terribly.

This was an unusually clear and succinct response that indicated in-depth understanding.

Penny, is it now fully clear to you how you learned to be sick to avoid school? *Yes, it is. It's pretty clear. My mother was a teacher. Yes, it is very clear.*

In a three-month, and follow-up interview, Penny reported hav-ing not been sick at all and expressed her delight in having sur-mounted her lifelong problem.

Mary – Subliminal Therapy by Telephone

Mary was a 50-something female who lived in a city in another state. Her presenting concern was a block that prevented her from doing what she knew she was capable of doing, academically and professionally. This concern evolved into the goal of eliminating the inappropriate anger she felt toward her husband. The following excerpt is from the third session.

Fred (her husband) seems to think things are fine unless I am upset.

Is there a better way to communicate your position to him? *Yes, by calm discussion and more speaking up.*

Centrum, do you agree with that conclusion? YES

Centrum, does any part of your mind disagree with that conclusion? YES, THREE

Centrum, are you in communication with all three of those parts? YES

Centrum, do you know what to do in this situation without assistance? YES And, Centrum, are you willing to do that now? YES Then please address each of those parts, one at a time, persuading each to your way of thinking. Let me know when you have done so by the word "complete". COMPLETE

Centrum, were you successful in all three cases? NO Were you successful with any of the parts? YES, TWO

Centrum, are you in communication with the third part? NO Are you willing to communicate with that part? YES Is the part willing to communicate with you? NO

Centrum, is the part willing to receive information under the condition that it is not required to reveal itself? NO

A "no" response at this point is very unusual.

Centrum, is the part well-intended? YES Is the part capable of learning? YES

Centrum, how old were you when that part came into existence? 2

Here, I have acted on a hunch.

Centrum, do you have the memory of that 2-year-old experience? NO

Here again, I acted on insight.

Mary, allow your mind to drift back in time, back in time to that take care of time when you were 2 years old and something happened that relates to the work you are doing now. *I have a picture of my mother and aunt being angry. I felt scared. I'm very little. I'm confused. I learned that that's what big people do.*

Since even Centrum did not have access to the memory, I decided to take advantage of her trance state to regress her to the experience. It is most unusual that Centrum would not have access to the memory.

Tell me, Mary, does the lesson you learned then still apply in your life now, as an adult? *No!*

Centrum, do you agree with your conscious opinion? YES

Centrum, is that third part now willing to communicate with you? YES Centrum, you know what to do. Please take care of it. COMPLETE Centrum, were you successful? YES

Centrum, since uncovering and resolving one issue can make it possible to identify another issue, I ask that you search to identify any remaining parts of your mind, that might continue to interfere with you doing what you know to do. Did you identify any remaining parts? YES, FIVE

This response indicates that she has conscious awareness of Centrum that is aside from my communications with Centrum.

I think there were ten. Centrum, is that accurate, were there ten parts? YES

Centrum, do you know what to do? YES Let me know when you have done so. COMPLETE Centrum, were you successful, with all ten parts? NO

Centrum, did you have difficulty with one or more of those parts? YES, FOUR Centrum, are you in communication with all four of those parts? YES

Centrum, do you disagree with the position taken by part number one? YES

As the guide, I needed to know the overall situation, so I asked.

Centrum, do you disagree with the position taken by part number two? NO

Centrum, do you disagree with the position taken by part number three? YES

Centrum, do you disagree with the position taken by part number four? NO

Centrum, please elevate to consciousness the position taken by number one. *It has to do with my ex-husband, who told me I'd never make it without him.*

A classic illustration of hypnosis at work. She bought it without questioning it – he was the authority in that situation, at that time.

Well, Mary, that might well have been true then. Is it true now? *It's no longer true.*

Centrum, do you agree with your conscious opinion? YES AND NO Well, Centrum, with what part do you disagree? FEAR AND WORKING HARD

I don't understand that. Centrum, please make it clear. *I feel like I'm making this up … You are not like your mother. You don't have to work so hard.*

Do you believe you can make it without your ex-husband? NO!

Mary, what is your conscious reaction to that? *Shit! I don't understand why my higher wisdom would think that. Although, it is hard to do things without someone.*

Mary, can you make it alone? *Yes, but barely so.*

Chapter VI

Typical Problems Encountered

Problems in using Subliminal Therapy are varied, yet they are almost always manageable. Problems may have to do with communications, motivations, resistance or misunderstanding. They may derive from subconscious processes or conscious opinions, and they may have to do with the therapist's skill or with rapport. Such problems do not surface often, yet must be resolved when they do surface.

Communication Problems

Conscious Opinions Expressed in Lieu of Responses from Centrum

Instead of relaying the communications from Centrum as instructed, patients will sometimes persist in responding with conscious opinions they "are sure" are the correct answers. This is the most common problem in the administration of ST, and I've expanded upon some effective means of resolving it here. If treatment is to proceed productively, the clinician must find an objective way to differentiate between these conscious opinions and the communications from Centrum. Usually, if the clinician points out to the patient that conscious opinion has not resolved the problem thus far, the patient becomes willing to conform to the Guiding Rule.

Yet, it is all too often true that the patient will slip into conscious responses, especially if there is a delay in the response from Centrum. Our conditioning from cultural experiences, i.e., to be in conscious control, seems to slip in. It is highly important that the therapist confront every suspected response, beginning at the onset of treatment. A few patients will persist in responding consciously, even in the face of confrontations that approach rudeness. In such instances, one of my favorite reactions is to say with appropriate sensitivity, *"I don't care what you think! I only care about what Centrum communicates!"* Most patients, however, will eventually conform reliably.

On occasion, I have found it necessary to even be rudely abrupt in convincing the patient to refrain from expressions of conscious opinion. *"I cannot see your chalkboard, and when you speak to me I cannot tell the difference between your conscious opinions and the communications from Centrum. You have been stating your conscious opinions, as you admit, and I have assumed they were from Centrum. We have been spinning wheels and wasting time, not to mention your money. PLEASE abide by that Golden Rule we have discussed so many times."*

Handling Delayed Responses

In general, Centrum's responses to questions and requests will be prompt, sometimes coming even before the question is completed. Sometimes, however, responses may be delayed to the extent that both patient and therapist are concerned that Centrum has abandoned the requested task and gone to sleep.

If the delay exceeds a minute or so, I will intervene with a question to Centrum such as, *"Centrum, are you still engaged in the task I requested?"* If the answer is "Yes", I will acknowledge the response and request that the patient be patient also. Only in rare cases have I needed to intervene with that question more than once during a long pause.

If the answer to the above question is "No", I will inquire if Centrum is willing to continue the work, essentially starting the protocol again. Alternatively, I might ask if Centrum needs assistance in completing the task. It is important to bear in mind that Centrum is not a source of infinite wisdom. Centrum too has limitations that must be respected, and your guidance and clinical judgment may be required to both guide and bridge the gap in Centrum's abilities.

Resistance to Change

In the course of all psychotherapy, resistance to change becomes the focus of treatment. In ST, with the exception of conscious resistance, resistance is understood to be the proactive action of one or more parts in the subconscious domain, parts that are resisting change because their beliefs are contrary to the goal of therapy. The task is to recondition these parts that have been 'locked in the past' such that they become aware of, and supportive of, the patient's present circumstances.

Conscious Resistance to Change

Conscious resistance to change may exist because of consciously recognized, conflicting interests and values. These issues are resolvable; however, they may require the clinician to participate in reaching a balance of the factors involved, concluding with the best compromise that can be reached. For example, giving up pain has an obvious benefit, yet doing so may mean less attention being paid to the person. The questions become: *"Which is of greater value to the patient?"* and *"Is compromise possible?"* The answers to these questions may be obvious to the therapist; however, the values of the therapist must remain outside the process. Pose those questions to the part, even if it seems redundant to do so.

Subconscious Resistance to Change

You will encounter resistance based on *subconscious* reasoning far more frequently than *conscious* resistance. After all, it is conscious motivation that brought the patient to therapy. Resistance from the subconscious domain will seldom appear rational to conscious reasoning; however, it is important to recognize that the reasoning *is* rational from the perspective of the resisting part. In a sense, you must initially join with that resisting part, communicating from its perspective, educating and persuading as necessary.

As in other cultures, in our culture we are taught to be in control, to get the information, to make a decision and to act on it. Yet, our actual ability to control ourselves comes into question. Who among us does not have some habit or engage in some behavior we wish were not part of our lives? In such instances, we subconsciously resist change even though we consciously desire it.

Manifestations of Subconscious Resistance

The patient's subjective, conscious experience of subconscious resistance can take many forms; however, it usually conforms to one of these three forms:

Interfering with, or preventing, communications from Centrum. The most common means of interfering is by preventing the patient from visualizing a chalkboard, closely followed by placing the chalkboard at such a distance that the patient is unable to read the words written thereon. Also, the image of the chalkboard might be distorted or fogged over. Some letters of the words may be missing and distraction in the form of physical activity is another means of interference. Patients have exhibited endless variations.

Parts unwilling or unable to communicate with Centrum. One of the most common actions by the therapist in the course of using ST is to request that Centrum establish communications with problematic parts. A resistant part may unilaterally refuse to communicate, requiring a deviation from the ideal steps of the decision tree. When this occurs, the therapist needs to persuade the part to communicate and this necessarily becomes the immediate focus of treatment.

If the resisting part is refusing to communicate with Centrum, ask Centrum if the part is willing "just to listen," without being required to expose itself. Assuming an affirmative answer, and it usually is, ask Centrum to communicate information about current reality *to* that part and to advise you when it has been accomplished. When so advised, ask if the part is now willing to communicate fully with Centrum to ensure mutual understanding between them. The answer will consistently be "Yes", and Centrum should then be requested to persuade the part to cooperate in the treatment.

Fabricating distracting scenarios. The human imagination knows no limits, and this seems to apply also to the abilities of the other parts of the mind. For the clinician, varied distractions of this sort can be the most frustrating form of resistance because there seems to be no objective way to detect their occurrence. Although seldom encountered, such fabrications often have a ring of truth about them that conforms with the content being addressed in the session. Detection becomes a challenge to the talents of the clinician.

Resolving Subconscious Resistance

When the therapist encounters barriers in the course of applying ST, these obstacles are manifestations of subconscious, conditioned beliefs that were, at one point in time – at that point when they were learned – logical and functional. The part of the mind representing such beliefs understands them as the *only* reality, and fear of the consequences of change is consistently the basis for subconscious resistance. One or more parts of the mind may strongly hold a resistant position and, by one means or another, each part must be persuaded to support, rather than resist, the goal of therapy if the goal is to be achieved.

If the resisting part is preventing or interfering with communication from Centrum by preventing the patient from visualizing a chalkboard, and you have not been successful in guiding Centrum to resolve the resistance, establish an alternate method of communication such as ideo-motor response. Using the alternate method, guide Centrum to identify, communicate with and educate the resisting part about the negative consequence of its resistance, thereby resolving the resistance and hopefully permitting return to the use of the chalkboard. If this is unsuccessful, assume that the resisting part is able to hear you directly and address the part in the second person. Patiently and comprehensively educate the part about current reality and the need for change. This may seem an awkward and foolish exercise at first; however, it is generally effective. Set your sense of feeling foolish aside and do it anyway; the results can make it worth the effort.

If the resisting part has led you astray by misinformation, ask if Centrum is capable of resolving the problem without assistance from you. If "Yes", request Centrum to do so. "No" implies that Centrum is in communication with the part and Centrum should be asked to persuade the part to cooperate with treatment, doing so by educating the part about current needs. If Centrum is not in communication with the part, reaffirm the willingness of Centrum to so communicate and begin the process anew.

Chapter VII

Research on the Efficacy of Subliminal Therapy

The author's experience with many hundreds of patients has indicated a high order of efficacy in the use of Subliminal Therapy, as have anecdotal reports from others who were trained in the technique. Inadequately controlled research was conducted in the early years and is reported below; however, it was not until 2008 that more meaningful measures of effectiveness were instituted. These measures will be described and the results reported.

Early Research

Subliminal Therapy was initially evaluated in 1977 by a review of the clinical records of forty-one patients, of random age and sex, who presented a total of 161 problems, including a wide variety of behavioral, somatic, emotional, phobic, and sexual concerns. I treated these patients on an individual basis in a private, clinical setting for an average of 6.2 hours each. All patients were treated for multiple presenting problems. Achievement of all therapeutic goals was self-reported a minimum of one-month post-treatment by thirteen of the patients (32 percent), and achievement of at least half of their therapeutic goals by an additional 17 (41 percent). These results are reported without claim of adequate research controls. The data were compiled, in some cases, months after the therapeutic work was done.

In 1978, a study was conducted in which three females were treated for hay fever using ST. Following three individual treatment sessions, two reported their symptoms had completely vanished, and the third reported an improvement of 35–40 percent.

The three sessions lasted an average of twenty-one minutes each, following initial introduction, history-taking and instruction, so that each subject was seen individually for an average of sixty-three minutes.

In early 1979, as a test of the theory that the therapist could successfully treat patients without knowing the nature of the presenting problem, five subjects were so treated. With the assistance of a colleague, I was given the first name of the subjects, and information as to whether they wished to eliminate some influence or to achieve something. I was made aware of their presenting goals only after the conclusion of the study. Four of the five successfully accomplished their goals.

Later in 1979, I conducted a pilot study in which a computerized version of Subliminal Therapy was employed in lieu of a human therapist. Five subjects presenting simple phobias were treated in a context that limited instructions to printed material, contact with the therapist being confined to logistic issues. Four of the five subjects reported successful elimination of their phobias. Two reported success during the first treatment session, one subject required two sessions, and the fourth required three. The duration of treatment sessions, i.e., interaction with the computer, was determined by the subject being treated and varied from seventeen minutes to forty-eight minutes.

Current Research

Beginning in August of 2008, I accumulated data to objectively evaluate the effectiveness and efficiency of ST. The data formalized in the following paragraphs were derived from patient-completed inventories obtained in my private practice in San Diego, California.

Methods

Subjects. The subjects of this study were all patients in my private practice. All eighty-two patients were adults with a mean age of 38 years, most of whom presented more than one problem. Thirty-five patients were male, forty-seven were female. Of the 156 problems reported here, sixty-two were presented by males and ninety-four were presented by females. Thirteen patients were excluded from the study because of incomplete treatment; they either terminated prematurely or were currently in treatment.

Procedure. In each case, the initial session was devoted to individual history and evaluation, and all subjects were instructed in the self-use of hypnosis. All were provided with a copy of *Subliminal Therapy: Utilizing the Unconscious Mind* (Yager, 1985), and were instructed to read it prior to the next appointment. Subjects were typically seen one or two times per week for one-hour sessions and all were treated by ST.

Data collection. Patients were asked to complete a brief inventory form at the initial session, again at the conclusion of treatment and (currently in execution) at a follow-up time period. The form used was a one-page inventory of the negative effects the presenting problem was having on the patient's life. The following questions were asked and the patient was requested to indicate the degree of effect by marking on a continuum representing "Not at all" to "Severe" that followed each question. In the event that more than one problem was presented, a separate form was used for each problem.

To what extent are the symptoms present in your life?
To what extent has the above problem interfered with your social life?
To what extent has the above problem interfered with your family life?
To what extent has the above problem interfered with your sexual life?
To what extent has the above problem interfered with your spiritual life?
To what extent has the above problem interfered with your memory?
To what extent has the above problem interfered with your sleep?

To what extent has the above problem interfered with your appetite?

To what extent has the above problem interfered with your work life?

To what extent has the above problem interfered with your ability to concentrate?

To what extent has the above problem been a cause of personal distress?

To what extent has the above problem caused you to feel depressed?

To what extent has the above problem caused you to feel anxious?

To what extent has the above problem caused physical problems?

To what extent has the above problem caused any other problem(s)?

If your response is affirmative, what is that problem?

Data processing. The data were quantified by marking each continuum to represent zero to ten, recording the value marked thereon, and averaging the scores. The averaged before-and-after scores were then evaluated using the effect size computation of Cohen's *d*.

Results

The results of the study are summarized in Table 1.

The diagnoses were obtained by DSM criteria. Expansion of the details of the data, in addition to newly added subjects, is available on the Subliminal Therapy Institute website, www.stii.us.

I have been asked if the extraordinary effectiveness of Subliminal Therapy might be due to my personal talents as a psychotherapist. In response, I say that while the training and personal attributes of the clinician are absolutely part of the equation, I cannot attribute such a high level of success to any therapist, no matter his or her talents.

Table 1 – Effectiveness of Subliminal Therapy

	Average treatment hours	Effect size Cohen's *d*	Average improvement	*n* Number of cases	*n* > 80%
Addiction	**2.1**		**94%**	**10**	**9**
Chemical	2.5	1.15	98%	3	3
Smoking	2.0	0.93	99%	4	4
Other	2.0	1.06	84%	3	2
Anxiety	**3.2**		**80%**	**57**	**39**
General Anxiety	4.2	0.26	87%	24	19
OCD	2.1	0.28	61%	17	5
Panic D	2.8	0.36	85%	12	9
Phobic D	1.5	0.39	82%	10	6
Mood	**3.0**		**82%**	**25**	**15**
Anger	2.0	0.37	83%	12	7
Depression	2.8	0.71	79%	4	3
Guilt	4.4	0.43	74%	8	4
Physical	**2.9**		**68%**	**31**	**19**
Asthma	2.0	1.57	84%	2	1
Gastro-intestinal	4.7	0.25	75%	3	1
Pain	2.5	0.33	75%	14	9
Weight	3.2	0.55	57%	3	0
Other	1.9	0.86	87%	9	6
Sexual	**7.8**		**97%**	**4**	**4**
Performance	21	1.84	93%	2	2
Vaginismus	5.0	2.00	100%	2	2
Sleep D	**2.9**	0.49	**82%**	**8**	**4**
Other	**2.9**	0.27	**86%**	**19**	**16**
Total				**156**	

Limitations of the Study

The data obtained in this study was derived exclusively from patients who were treated by the author in his private practice. Therefore, the data may not accurately represent the results of treatment by Subliminal Therapy if conducted by others.

While some follow-up data is available, which thus far confirms the results reported above, there has not yet been adequate follow-up to fully validate the results.

Efficacy of Other Therapies

A search was conducted to identify studies that would provide data with which to compare the efficacy of ST with other protocols. Only a few of the studies identified included objective data; most were reported in verbal terms with expressions such as "significantly significant improvement". Table 2 shows the results of those studies that reported data in a comparable form, and serves to provide data for the comparison.

Table 2 – Success Rates of Other Therapies

Study	Results
As quoted in Pigott et al., Turner et al. (2008) compared the effect size derived from the FDA repository to that from 51 published studies on antidepressant treatment.	Weighted means effect sizes FDA data set 0.31 Published studies 0.41
Roy-Byrne et al. (2004) conducted a trial of CBT vs. medications for panic disorder involving 6 treatment sessions with up to 6 follow-up sessions.	At 3 months: CBT was 46% vs. medications at 27%, $n = 232$ At 12 months: CBT was 63% vs. medications at 38%
Rector et al. (2009) examined the efficacy of CBT for OCD in patients with MDD.	$F = 12.33$, $df = 1.27$, $P = 0.002$, $d = 0.77$ $n = 27$

Table 2 (continued)

Study	Results		
Norton & Price (2007) conducted a meta-analytic review of 108 trials of CBT across the anxiety disorders.		**Pre-Post**	**Post-FU**
	PD/A	1.37 (6)	0.08 (5)
	SAD	1.03 (3)	0.21 (3)
	OCD	1.16 (7)	0.08 (3)
	GAD	2.06 (6)	0.29 (5)
	PTSD	2.23 (3)	0.54 (3)
	Overall	1.67	0.22
Hendricks et al. (2008) examined the efficacy of CBT for late-life anxiety disorders.	*SMD* = –0.51 (95% *CI*: –0.81), *P* < 0.001 Seven papers reviewed with *n* = 297		
Rezvan et al. (2008) compared the effectiveness of CBT with CBT and interpersonal therapy combined in the treatment of generalized anxiety disorder.	CBT Cohen's *d* = 2.700, *r* = 0.804, *n* = 36 CBT + IPT Cohen's *d* = 2.848, *r* = 0.818 Control Cohen's *d* = 1.315, *r* = 0.549		
Hynninen et al. (2010) examined the effect of CBT in groups for co-morbid, clinically significant anxiety and depression on COPD outpatients.	Anxiety effect size = 1.1, *n* = 26 Depression effect size = 0.9		
Keller et al. (2000) compared nefazodone with CBT and the combination of nefazodone plus CBT in the treatment of chronic depression.	Nefazodone 55%, *n* = 681 CBT 52% Combination 85%		
Coventry and Gellaty (2007) looked at CBT, given with exercise training and education, in the treatment of moderate anxiety and depression in COPD patients.	Anxiety –21.39 (95% Cls –22.19, –20.59) Depression –20.86 (95% Cls –21.61, –20.11)		

Note: Data on length of treatment by CBT was particularly difficult to identify. As quoted by Gale Thompson on *Healthline:* "Like behavior therapy, cognitive behavior therapy tends to be short-term (often between 10 and 20 sessions)". See www.healthline.com/galecontent/cognitive-behavior-therapy#cognitivebehaviortherapy.

Table 3 – Success Rates of Eye Movement Desensitization Reprocessing

Study	Results		
Ahmad and Sundelin-Wahlsten (2007) conducted a study of the effectiveness of EMDR on children diagnosed with PTSD. They found that EMDR mostly improved re-experiencing symptoms.	PTSD-related: 0.22 PTSD non-related: 0.06 Re-experiencing: 0.40 Avoidance: 0.21 Hyper-arousal: 0.01		
Bloomgarden and Calogero (2008) examined the short- and long-term effects of EMDR in a residential eating disorders population by comparing SRT treatment with SRT+EMDR; they found that SRT+EMDR was more effective at post-treatment and subsequent follow-ups, and concluded that "EMDR may be used to treat specific aspects of negative body image in conjunction with SRT."	Earliest body image Worst body image Most recent body image	**Pre-Tx** 0.008 0.001 0.004	**Post-Tx** 0.382 (Cohen's *d*) 0.362 0.211
Edmond et al. (1999) conducted a randomized experimental evaluation and found support for the effectiveness of EMDR in reducing trauma symptoms among adult female survivors of childhood sexual abuse.	– MANOVA (at follow-up) 1.29 (Cohen's *d*) – STAI (at follow-up) 1.02 – BI (at follow-up) 1.08		
Grainger et al. (1997) conducted an empirical study of the effectiveness of EMDR for traumatic symptoms in survivors of Hurricane Andrew. They found that EMDR may have more efficacy and efficiency than some other treatments.	SUDs A paired-comparison yielded $t(28) = 12.08$, $p < 0.001$	**Pre-Tx** 7.72 (SD = 1.58)	**Post-Tx** 1.93 (SD = 2.05)
Ironson et al. (2002) conducted a study on the efficacy of EMDR in treating PTSD; they found that EMDR was an effective treatment.	PTSD BDI	*t* 3.36 4.25	*p* 0.008 0.001

Table 3 (continued)

Study	Results				
Jaberghaderi et al. (2004) conducted a study comparing CBT and EMDR for effectiveness in treating sexual abuse victims; they found that "EMDR was significantly more efficient, with large effect sizes on each outcome."		**CBT**	**EMDR**		
	CROPS:	$d = 1.1$	$d = 2.8$ (Cohen's d)		
	PROPS:	$d = 1.1$	$d = 1.8$		
	RUTTER:	$d = 0.72$	$d = 0.71$		

Study	Results				
Puffer et al. (1998) in a study measuring the effectiveness of EMDR treatment on trauma patients, found that "all measures showed statistically significant treatment effects in the desired direction," and "the measures which focused directly on the traumatic memory (IES, SUDS, VoC) showed a stronger response to the EMDR treatment than did the CMAS."		**M**	**SD**	t	p
	CMAS	−6.2	8.8	3.2	0.005
	IES	−24.8	17.4	6.4	0.0001
	SUDS	−8.8	1.8	21.7	0.0001
	VoC	+5.2	1.3	17	0.0001
	"p" values are 2-tailed and reflect the difference between the final pre-treatment assessment and the 1–3 month follow-up.				

Study	Results		
Scheck et al. (1998) conducted a study to measure the efficacy of EMDR in treating traumatized patients. In comparison with AL (Active Listening) treatment, they found "significant improvement for both groups and significantly greater pre-post change for EMDR-treated participants. Pre-post effect sizes for the EMDR group averaged 1.56 compared to 0.65 for the AL group. Despite treatment brevity, the post-treatment outcome variable means of EMDR-treated participants compared favorably with non-patient or successfully treated norm groups on all measures."		**AL**	**EMDR**
	BECK:	$d = 0.67$	$d = 1.44$ (Cohen's d)
	STATE:	$d = 0.63$	$d = 1.65$
	PENN:	$d = 0.77$	$d = 1.49$
	IES:	$d = 0.52$	$d = 2.09$
	TCS:	$d = 0.66$	$d = 1.15$

Conclusions

Subliminal Therapy demonstrates an unusually high effect size over an unusually wide range of presenting problems, physical as well as mental, in a shorter time than CBT or medications. ST demonstrated an overall effect size of 2.11 with CBT demonstrating 1.41 and EMDR demonstrating 1.55 in available meta-analyses. ST is significantly more efficacious than both CBT and EMDR in terms of effectiveness, and in efficiency as well.

Chapter VIII

The Subliminal Therapy Institute, Inc.

Formation

The Subliminal Therapy Institute, Inc. (STI, Inc.) established in 2009 as a non-profit, California 501(c)(3) corporation and is qualified as a non-profit corporation by the Federal Government.

Objectives

- To provide training and certification of training in the clinical use of Subliminal Therapy to licensed health-care professionals.

- To provide research opportunities to test and expand the scope of applications of Subliminal Therapy.

- To educate the public about the benefits of Subliminal Therapy.

Training and Certification in Subliminal Therapy

I am sometime asked about available training in Subliminal Therapy. How long does it take to become proficient? Can I ethically use ST before I have become fully proficient? Is there certification in ST? Where can I obtain training?

Training

In answer to such questions as those above, formal, structured training in ST is available through STI, Inc. For those able to attend training is San Diego, this training includes opportunities to observe other clinicians who are conducting research in the clinical efficacy of ST, access to the library of the Institute that includes numerous DVDs of demonstrations, supervised practice of the principles of ST and the opportunity to become certified in its use.

On a more pragmatic level, for many clinicians, training is available via workshops and a planned series of trainings to be delivered across the country. These trainings can be augmented by your study of DVDs of recorded sessions, available from the Institute at www.stii.us. If you are interested to setting up a group training in your area, contact me at doc@docyager.com.

Once the concepts of ST have been integrated, and the clinician has been trained to think in the philosophy of ST, proficiency can be expected with as little as ten to twenty hours of practice in its application. And, as with all things, the longer you use it, the more proficient you become. I am better at it today than I was a year ago, even after almost forty years of practice.

Certification

Licensed clinicians may be certified in Subliminal Therapy *only* by the Subliminal Therapy Institute, Inc. The qualifications and training for this certification, and its responsibilities and privileges are as follows:

Qualifications:

- Applicant must be *licensed* as a health-care clinician in the state of his or her practice.

- Applicant must hold membership in a professional organization commensurate with license.

Training:

- Training may be completed in the facilities of STI, Inc., or elsewhere under the supervision of a clinician who has been certified by STI, Inc. In the latter case, formal recommendation to STI, Inc., by a certified clinician will qualify the applicant to take the written examination offered by STI, Inc., and the demonstration of proficiency requirement as described below must be met to the satisfaction of the recommending clinician.

- A syllabus of training materials will be provided to the applicant and the applicant must be familiar with that material to be able to pass the certification test.

- Applicant must have observed a minimum of fifteen hours of the application of Subliminal Therapy by other clinicians prior to taking the certification test.

Proof of competency:

- Applicant must pass a certification test consisting of 100 computer-generated questions as provided by STI, Inc., with a minimum score of 98 percent. The contents of this test will be randomly selected for each administration of the test from the list of training questions in the syllabus. A fee will be payable for each administration of the test and the applicant will be permitted to retake the test as many times as desired.

- Following passing of the certification test, applicant must demonstrate proficiency in using Subliminal Therapy by performing psychotherapy for a minimum of five hours under the direct supervision of a certified clinician. The supervising clinician must formally certify that the applicant has satisfactorily demonstrated proficiency.

Obligations:

- It is an obligation of a certified person to encourage the use of Subliminal Therapy in those applications where it is appropriate to do so.

- It is an obligation of a certified person to train other clinicians who are interested in using Subliminal Therapy.

Privileges:

- Your name, links and related data will be posted on the website of the Institute.

- You will be eligible for referrals from the Institute.

- You will have authorization to publicize your certification in any responsible way.

- You will have access to consultants associated with STI, Inc.

- You will have access to restricted information on the website of the Institute.

- As opportunity and availability coincide, you will have authority to teach others how to use Subliminal Therapy.

Promotion of Subliminal Therapy

Since conceiving Subliminal Therapy in 1974, I have been promoting its use within the professional communities of medicine and psychology. After many presentations, workshops and classes, I have concluded that another approach is also required.

Having the data to support claims of success has been of some help in getting professional attention; however, even with the data, I observe only minimal use outside of my private practice. It seems that professionals of all disciplines are trained in the techniques of tradition and lack motivation to expand their capabilities.

Therefore, I have concluded that I must publicize the technique to the extent that the public will demand the availability of Subliminal Therapy. The professions will then respond, if motivated only by economics. To this end, I formed the Subliminal Therapy Institute, Inc. in 2009, with the threefold objectives of research, training and promotion. Formal papers and training for the professions will continue, but with the added emphasis on public exposure.

Subliminal Therapy Institute, Inc.
3737 Moraga Ave. Suite A-203
San Diego CA 92117

Website: www.stii.us

Chapter IX

Other Considerations

The Self-Use of Subliminal Therapy

Patients sometimes ask about the self-use of Subliminal Therapy. I encourage their inquiry and suggest they explore its possibilities. Yet I am aware of an intrinsic limitation to their doing so: the simple fact that we seem incapable of being objective about ourselves. We usually need another person to provide that objectivity.

Yet, there are some things we *can* do for ourselves, and there is nothing to be lost in going for it. Patients can objectively communicate with Centrum themselves without assistance. Using Subliminal Therapy, my patients have reported success in maintaining discipline in their behavior, uncovering the roots of problems that had been addressed in other therapy techniques and identifying influences that had not been consciously recognized.

Problems to Expect

- Shifting back and forth between the roles of being the guide of the process and the one seeking solution can be awkward.

- If questions arise, no assistance is immediately available.

- Questions or misgivings about accepting communications from Centrum as being valid are possible and answers are not available.

- Maintaining focus of attention on the goal, when required to shift back and forth between the roles of patient and guide, can be a problem if you become too involved in the process or content of the work, thereby losing sight of the goal to be accomplished.

How to be Effective

- Discipline your mind to define the first, *general objectives* of your efforts. For example, *"Be happy,"* or *"Become more acceptable to others,"* or *"Save my marriage."*

- Define one or more *specific* goals that are required to achieve each general objective. For example, *"Eliminate my compulsive behavior,"* or *"Stop my nagging behavior,"* or *"Sleep all night, every night."* Make a list of your goals so the process can flow smoothly, minimizing the problem of shifting back and forth.

- Define a reliable means of perceiving communications from Centrum, such as a chalkboard, computer screen or inner voice.

- Establish communication with Centrum.

- Inquire if Centrum agrees with your goal and is willing to support it. If not, refer to the decision-tree format as presented in Appendix A for guidance.

- Ask Centrum to accomplish all tasks that Centrum can accomplish without assistance.

- Progress through the decision-tree format as presented in Appendix A.

An Example

My wife uses ST by first identifying her objective, and then by narrowing the field of inquiry about impediments to her goal, moving from general questions to specific questions to achieve conscious understanding of the cause of the problem. Then she achieves resolution by re-decision or reframing that which she learned. She may or may not turn the task of accomplishment over to Centrum. Examples of general questions would be, "Does it have to do with family/work/home/etc.?" The next generation of questions might include, "Does it have to do with Ed?" The next might be, "What did he do?" Notice that her questions are not limited to yes/no responses; they are leading in nature, requiring analytic thought on the part of Centrum, as well as elaboration in responding.

My Wife's Self-Reported Case History

Three weeks before my son was born, I was involved in a car accident. The other person ran a stop sign and I crashed into her car – head on. When my son was 4 months old, he had to have life and death surgery. Shortly after that my father-in-law died.

I began having migraine headaches. They were incredibly debilitating. I had read so much about becoming dependent on prescription drugs that I refused to take anything stronger than Tylenol. Plus, I had a doctor who gave me 'permission' to have migraines by saying, "With all you've been through in the past few months it's no wonder you have headaches."

I suffered through the headaches for a couple of years, and then in the process of therapy, I discovered the real reason behind the headaches – it was to get attention. With that information, I decided to find another way to get attention, and the headaches disappeared for several years. The therapeutic technique that led me to the discovery of the actual cause of the headaches was Subliminal Therapy. My communication path to Centrum was, at the time, with a pendulum.

Then my marriage fell apart and the migraines returned. It turns out that when your head hurts that bad you can't think about all the scary things that are happening in your life. So I continued having good days and bad days. At the same time my marriage was breaking up, I took a test to become a computer programmer. And I, who had never even seen a computer (this was in the time before PCs), passed the test.

So, in a very short period of time, I got divorced, moved with my children to a new part of the city and started a new career. And guess what? Migraines! I was sure the cause was directly related to the new career, which was incredibly stressful. I was prepared to quit my job and go back to my former career, which was really just a job and not a career.

However, before I actually quit, I decided I should check with Centrum to be sure it was the job causing the headaches. I sat down at the table with my pendulum and began to ask a series of yes/no questions. Did Centrum know the cause? Was it home? Was it work? There was great resistance to getting to the real issue. As I started working with the pendulum, I became so sleepy that I would literally fall asleep sitting up waiting for the answer. I recognized this as resistance, so I decided I could take the pendulum and sit in the bathtub. Surely I wouldn't fall asleep in the tub. And it worked – no sleeping in the bathtub. I got the hiccoughs instead. Pendulums don't work with hiccoughs at all!

Resistance doesn't get much stronger than that. And I was still convinced that the only thing for me to do about the migraines was to quit my job. Finally, after some serious conversation with Centrum about my conscious desire to work through this issue, I got through the resistance and could work with the pendulum once more.

Again, I started with the yes/no questions:

> Was it work? No
> Was it home? Yes
> Was it the children? Yes
> … and on and on.

After a lot of struggling to find the right questions, I got to the root of the problem – I was feeling guilty about getting divorced and taking the children away from their father. Knowing that this was really the issue had two benefits:

1. I didn't quit the new job which ultimately turned into a successful career for me.

2. I had the opportunity to deal with the real problem (guilt) and the migraines stopped.

Actually, there was a third benefit. I learned that my conscious perceptions are not always accurate and that taking time to find the real cause/truth is always worth the time. I have since become proficient with ideo-motor response. I have a "Yes" finger and a "No" finger. When I'm struggling but don't exactly know why, I start with the yes/no questions, until I get to the truth. Knowing the truth doesn't always fix the problem, but at least I'm focused on the real problem, not wasting time with something else.

Suggestions for the Self-Use of Subliminal Therapy

- To become effective in self-hypnosis, an auto-suggestion (i.e., a suggestion to oneself) must be acceptable both consciously and subconsciously. Ask Centrum if the suggestion is acceptable, rather than just assuming it is.

- In the event a suggestion is not acceptable, ask Centrum to do what is necessary to make it so. Then ask Centrum if it has been accomplished.

Note: This does not guarantee accomplishment; Centrum may disagree with your conscious opinion. If so, in following the protocol you might find out why, and if Centrum does disagree, you might be able to convince Centrum that your way of thinking is the right way by talking to Centrum as if it were another person. Present your case as if you were in a courtroom.

- If interested, you might be able to find out why the suggestion for conscious awareness was not acceptable. Interact with Centrum and ask.

- If you are in a situation where you are bored, ask Centrum to make time go by quickly.

- Request support from Centrum in unusual and perhaps unexpected circumstances; for example, when you must make a formal presentation or must deliver an unwelcome message.

- By interacting with Centrum, you might be able to:

1. Eliminate an undesired behavior by learning about its roots and making a different decision than you made the first time.

2. Control undesired eating behavior by learning about its roots and making a different decision than you made the first time.

3. Control exaggerated anger by learning how you acquired it and making a different decision than you made the first time.

4. Control anxiety, depression, irritable bowel syndrome and the common cold by learning about its cause and making a different decision than you made the first time.

5. Regain a sense of personal power by learning how you lost it and making a different decision than you initially made when you lost it.

As another example of self-use: My wife gets a rash under her wedding ring when she is irritated with me about something. By playing Twenty Questions with Centrum, she is able to identify the cause of her irritation and resolve it either by correcting it, changing her perception about it or discussing it with me to find a mutually workable solution.

Subliminal Therapy by Telephone

On a few occasions, I have interacted with patients by telephone in guiding them through the protocol of Subliminal Therapy. In each instance, the treatment flowed well and was successful, yet there are certain differences in conducting the process when there are no visual cues to guide you. For example, the signs of trance (physical relaxation, absence of volitional movement, etc.) are not available. Truthfully, there is not a great deal of difference between telephone and office situations. Even in the office, there are only minimal cues of value; the patient is probably in trance, displaying no visually perceivable actions. You might close your eyes, and it would be the same as communicating by telephone.

Comparing Subliminal Therapy with Direct Hypnotic Suggestions

From one perspective, comparing Subliminal Therapy with direct (or even indirect) hypnotic suggestion is like comparing patient empowerment with patient disempowerment. In ST, patients are taught to utilize their own history and abilities to resolve the problem. In the use of direct suggestion, the patient is influenced by the opinions and biases of the clinician.

I believe the patient is best served when the clinician is least involved in the *content* of the work. The clinician cannot possibly know and understand all of the factors involved in the patient's condition. Therefore, opinions held by the clinician retain the possibility of inappropriately biasing or misdirecting the work of therapy.

The Use of a Computer in Lieu of a Therapist

Those familiar with computer technology will recognize that you can easily program the decision-tree format of the flow charts for computer use. As mentioned in Chapter VI, I demonstrated this use of ST employing a much less sophisticated decision tree than is provided in this book and with a surprisingly successful outcome. It is my intention to pursue this application of ST, and I have begun research on this undertaking.

Premature Withdrawal from Treatment

Patients often frustrate me by being satisfied with only *improvement* of their symptoms, whereas I seek *cure*. They sometimes pull away from treatment before attaining a full cure, stating they had achieved what they needed to achieve. My concern is that they may have only experienced a temporary remission and that recurrence is likely.

Duration of Treatment

Even after having accomplished their goal, patients occasionally question the possibility of completing treatment of long-term problems in such a brief period of time. When this question arises, I respond by pointing out that they learned the problem in a very brief period of time, perhaps in just a second or so. If conditioning can occur in that time, why cannot reconditioning occur in a similar amount of time?

When Using Ideo-Motor Responses

Ask the patient to speak the answers aloud as they perceive them to avoid your having to watch the fingers. However, if the patient is unaware of the finger motions, as is sometimes the case, you must watch the fingers!

A Legitimate Question

The question is sometimes asked: If Centrum has the ability to think, as I can consciously, why is it necessary to use ST at all? Why doesn't Centrum just take care of things?

The answer is that Centrum lacks the motivation to act (as do all parts in the subconscious domain). As incongruous as this may seem, it is consistently true; Centrum is rarely, if ever, proactive. On the other hand, Centrum is consistently willing to cooperate in the patient's recovery when appropriately guided.

When Symptoms Recur

You may assume the problem has been articulated, the cause identified and all identifiable parts have been educated appropriately at the last treatment session. Also, you may assume Centrum has indicated completion of the task, and the patient has indicated satisfaction that the work is complete. Yet, the patient calls a day or so later, reporting a continuation of one or more of the symptoms addressed and blaming himself for the 'failure' of the process. What to do?

Reaffirm what you know to be true, that the recurrence only means that the work is not complete, not that "it didn't work" or that the patient is a failure. The fire may appear to be out, yet there may be an unseen ember waiting to flare up. Persuade the patient to continue treatment, and do everything possible to counter the perception of failure. Point out that it doesn't mean the work was a failure, rather it means it is not complete. It is wise to make this point before the end of the last session.

When Centrum Responds in the First Person

Occasionally, you will have the good fortune to work with a patient whose Centrum responds orally and with eloquence. The patient will likely be of elevated IQ, inquisitive and openly involved at a conscious level. After the stage has been set, and communications with Centrum established, you may hear responses that sound suspiciously like conscious responses; they may be fully articulated and yet, when confronted, the patient convincingly assures you of their having come from Centrum. In such situations, you will be able to carry on a conversation with Centrum, much as you would with another person, and progress will be surprisingly rapid.

As an aside comment, be aware that, from patient to patient, Centrum can be of different gender than the patient and hold very different values and strengths. Moreover, these elements can change over time – yes, even gender.

When the Patient Has Compromised IQ

Subliminal Therapy is contra-indicated in all cases in which mental retardation is apparent and may be contra-indicated in cases of limited intelligence. The degree to which this is true has not been determined, therefore, clinical judgment must apply.

When the Patient is Consciously Confused

In a few cases, patients are consciously confused by the process of ST, wanting to understand what has been happening in their own minds. They may be resistant to continuing the process because of their need for conscious understanding. Requests to Centrum to provide the consciously desired information to the conscious satisfaction of the patient is usually adequate in these cases.

When the Patient Wants to Remember the Content – and Doesn't

It is not unusual for Centrum to do the work of therapy without there being conscious awareness of what is happening, and then also deny conscious awareness after completion of the protocol, presumably to protect the patient from the trauma of remembering some upsetting event. Some patients are okay with this situation, not really caring about knowing as long as the problem is resolved. Other patients really want to know and may be insistent about it.

If your decision is to pursue conscious awareness, first, determine if it is Centrum or some other part that objects to the memory becoming conscious. Then guide the patient to express his/her conscious opinion to the resisting part, doing so in the form of verbalization of the reason for wanting the information and while the objecting part is listening. If the patient can convince the objecting part to reveal the information, so much the better. If not, perhaps Centrum can convince the patient of the need for secrecy.

Centrum's Apparent Limits

If Centrum is requested to complete a task without assistance, such as to work without assistance between sessions, you will probably obtain agreement to do so; however, it is most often true that it does not happen. I have never understood this, but it seems that essentially all constructive work must be completed during the treatment session. There have been exceptions to this statement, but they are not common. And yet, to contradict this picture, there is indication that Centrum can be proactive if the stage is properly set, and if motivation to act is inspired in Centrum. Such motivation, of course, can come only from the conscious values of the patient; the subjective opinions and values of the therapist carry little weight.

Treating the Cause vs. Treating the Symptom

I believe the analytic approach to therapy is indicated in any case where the problem is psychogenic or where psychogenesis may play a role. Of course, the immediate clinical problem lies in differentiating between psychogenesis and other causes, and here again, the analytic approach can be used to aid in making that differentiation.

To illustrate my understanding of the way in which we function, consider the following examples: A disorder of the immune system is manifested as chemical changes in the body that, in general, can be identified. Yet, we can say the same thing about depression. I maintain that what we call depression is simply a conditioned response that causes the chemical imbalance, not the other way around, and the same principle of genesis applies in behavior and emotional problems. Can we not say the same about an immune disorder? My preferred course in treating depression is to focus on the cause, and that cause is almost never recognized consciously, even though it is common for the patient to consciously believe it is. Patients often express surprise when they learn the true cause and delight to find the presenting problem is no longer present.

So we may move from a *cause* (some life event) to a response that is a physical manifestation of the cause (such as malfunction of digestion), that in turn may be diagnosed as a physical *illness* (such as IBS), especially if the physical manifestation is chronic. This flow of events is commonly evident. The physiological explanation for this sequence is also clear: it is based in the action of smooth muscle that is, in turn, controlled by subconscious process.

A study of the functions of smooth muscle provides valuable information. Not only are the vital functions of life activated by smooth muscle (such as digestion, respiration, regulation of the pattern of blood flow in the body, etc.), so also are the glands themselves. Since this is established fact, and this musculature is controlled by subconscious process, is it surprising that dysfunction would occur in reaction to negative emotion? Moreover, the action of smooth muscle is evident in every bodily function, without exception to my knowledge.

I believe our role as therapists is to empower the patient by teaching skills the patient can use to correct their own problems, then guide them to use those skills. Teaching them to rationally utilize their higher level abilities, even though they had heretofore been unknown to them, seems to me to be an effective way to do so, and Subliminal Therapy is the most effective way I know to do that.

When Not To Use Subliminal Therapy

Subliminal Therapy is clearly contra-indicated when the problem is a broken bone, gushing blood or a heart attack. As is true for all psychological treatment, it is also contra-indicated if the patient is in denial of valid need for medical care and when the patient fears the consequence of medical attention (for example, if the patient fears "it might be cancer") and is seeking substitute care. On the other hand, it would be entirely appropriate to use ST to remove a psychological barrier to seeking medical care.

Subliminal Therapy will not work for everyone. Insistence on its use with a given patient could also be contra-indicated if the patient is unable to embrace the concepts of ST or if he seems incapable of communicating with Centrum.

The Future of Subliminal Therapy

Although the essential precepts of ST have remained constant during the thirty-plus years of development, it has evolved into an increasingly efficient and effective protocol. I anticipate it will continue to evolve, especially as new clinicians become involved, using their creative abilities. Thus far, it has been pretty much a one-man show. I conceived ST and have developed it into its present form. It is time now for others to assume an active role.

I anticipate the development of more ingenious ways to communicate with Centrum, which will permit wide usage of the computer therapist model and improved efficiency in general. Different and improved protocols are to be expected and a widening of the field of application will result, including innovations that are beyond my ability to even imagine.

One area of potential high value for the use of ST is in treating addictions. In all addictive situations, including addiction to street drugs, there is a psychological component that is at least as powerful as the chemical aspect. The physical symptoms of addiction – withdrawal and tolerance in particular – fade with time during abstinence. In the case of smoking tobacco, it is in the order of a week; in the case of heroin, it is many months. Yet, the addictive properties of the psychological addiction can last a lifetime. It is clear to me that the psychological aspect must be addressed if resolution of the addiction is to be achieved.

Another area of exceedingly high potential value is in the treatment of chronic pain. Based on the cases I have treated to date, it seems that psychological elements are not just major factors, they can be primary factors. Clearly, ST is the treatment of choice. At least to the extent of reducing pain, it has been effective in every case I have treated thus far. The case transcription *Tom: A Case of Pain from a Spinal Cord Injury* is illustrative of this principle. It seems so often true that pain, which starts as physical, mutates by related experiences to become psychogenic.

Appendix A: Flow Charts

In this Appendix, flow charts are offered as general guidelines for your use, especially while you are learning the process. In addition to the flow charts, suggested verbal content of each step of the charts is provided. Each numbered statement/question that appears on the Chart is accompanied by possible answers, with the number of the next step to take corresponding to that answer.

Unplanned deviations from the flow of therapy presented here can be expected as you interact with patients. I suggest you use your creative ability to guide the process back to the path of the charts, asking appropriate questions to resolve the interfering issues.

It is important to recognize that the path of the flow of the process defined in these guidelines is not the only path. This pathway will "work" in a large percentage of cases, but other pathways will be required in other cases. I believe the most significant element of Subliminal Therapy is the unique, direct, pragmatic and rational communication with Centrum that takes place. Engage that capacity of the patient's mind in a logical progression of steps and good outcome will follow.

The Basic Flow Chart

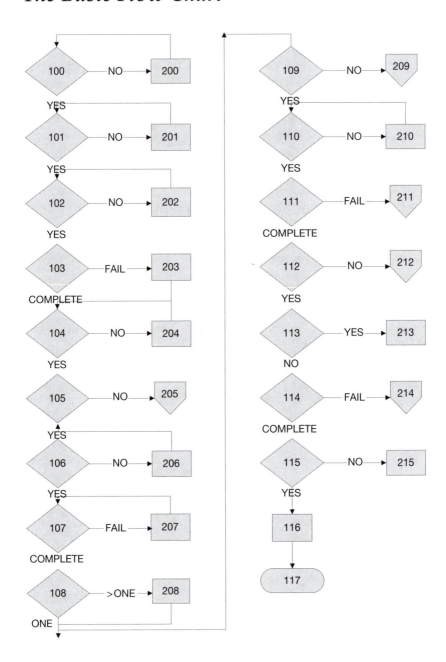

The Extended Flow Chart

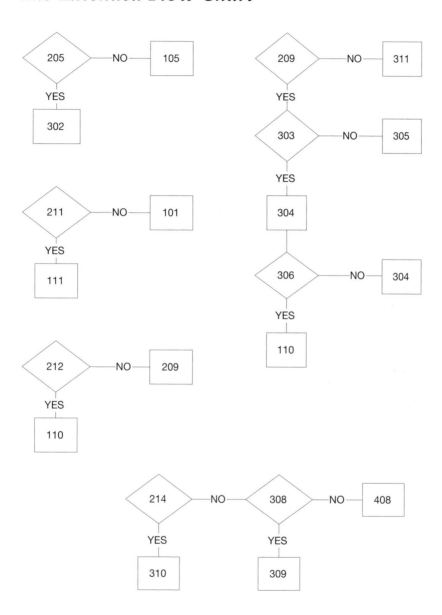

Verbal Content for the Steps on the Flow Charts

Note that the flow is addressed to the problem of asthma for convenience in presentation.

100 SERIES

100   Having set the stage to begin the process of Subliminal Therapy, you will now begin to follow the flow charts. Since you are advised to avoid assumptions, ensure that Centrum is aware of the conscious goal by asking. Do not assume Centrum is aware. Request that Centrum respond by writing the answer on the chalkboard.

Asking Centrum to indicate completion by writing the work "complete" following the first half-dozen steps of the process may make it unnecessary to repeatedly ask for the chalkboard response at the end of succeeding steps; the responses will come without the request.

Centrum, are you aware of your conscious desire/concern regarding the asthma? Please respond by writing your answer on the chalkboard.   Y – 101
                                                                                         N – 200

101   It is wise to ensure that Centrum is willing to be involved in the process. And if there is a negative response, it will be necessary to persuade Centrum to be involved. Here, your talents as a clinician come into play; however, it is rare that Centrum is not cooperative.

Centrum, are you willing to cooperate in this effort, to do some work as I guide you and teach you how, to accomplish your conscious goal?   Y – 102
                                                                                         N – 201

102   Ask Centrum to complete the investigation as comprehensively as possible with the objective of Centrum achieving as complete an understanding as is possible at this time, and to indicate completion of the task by writing the work "complete" on the chalkboard.

Centrum, please investigate this issue. Review memories of events that may have had something to do with it and communicate with those parts that are involved. The objective, Centrum, is for you to understand how asthma became part of your life. Centrum, is my request clear to you?   Y – 103
                                                                                         N – 202

103	*Centrum, please complete that task as comprehensively as is possible at this time and let me know when you have done so, to the limit of your ability, by writing the word "complete" on the chalkboard.*	C – 104 F – 203

104   Again, make no assumptions. Ask Centrum if the investigation produced understanding of the cause of the problem. If not, you must approach the process in a way that will ensure the development of Centrum's understanding.

	Centrum, do you now understand the cause of the asthma, how it came to be a part of your life and why it has continued?	Y – 105 N – 204

105   Ask Centrum if the asthma is being caused by one or more parts of the mind. If more than one, you must guide Centrum to interact with each part independently, one at a time, through Step 109 of the sequence.

	Centrum, is asthma being caused by the action of one or more parts of your mind?	Y – 106 N – 205

106	*Centrum, I will now ask that you identify the part, or parts if there are more than one, of your mind that are actively causing the asthma so that you will be able to communicate with them. Centrum, is that purpose clear to you?*	Y – 107 N – 206

107	*Centrum, please identify the part, or parts, and let me know when you have completed the task by writing the word "complete" on the chalkboard.*	C – 108 F – 207

108   Ask Centrum how many parts are actively involved in causing the asthma to occur, or in interfering or preventing the goal from being accomplished.

	Centrum, how many such parts are actively causing the asthma?	1 – 109 >1 – 208

109   Centrum may or may not be in communication with this particular part. You must ask.

	Centrum, are you in communication with that part?	Y – 110 N – 209

110   Explain to Centrum that the part is stuck in time, aware only of the information available at the time it was formed, and that it is in ignorance of present reality. Explain Centrum's job as being that of educating the part about present reality, thereby becoming aware of present life situations, values, needs, etc.

> *Centrum, please communicate with that part in the*
> *following way: First, please listen to the part. Find out*
> *what the part believes and why it believes what it believes.*
> *Then, Centrum, communicate to that part information*
> *about present reality. Centrum, that part is stuck in time*
> *at that time when it came into being, knowing only what*
> *it knew then, in ignorance of your life as it is now. Educate*
> *that part, Centrum, about present needs, values and life*
> *situation. Persuade that part to your way of thinking.* Y – 111
> *Centrum, is my request clear to you?* N – 210

111   Then, Centrum, please accomplish that task to the limit of
      your ability and let me know when you have done so by   C – 112
      writing the word "complete" on the chalkboard.   F – 211

112   Avoid assuming success. Ask!

      Centrum, did you succeed in that task?   Y – 113
                                                               N – 212

113   It is possible that Centrum accomplished more than you
      requested, or may have identified other active parts.

      Centrum, please search to identify any remaining part
      of your mind that may still be in a position to cause the
      asthma to continue. Is one or more parts of your mind still
      active in any way, for any reason, that might cause the N – 114
      asthma to recur in your life?   Y – 109

114   The patient may strongly desire conscious awareness of the
      work just completed, may be indifferent, or may not want to
      be aware. Nevertheless, conscious awareness does seem to
      afford value to the process and, unless there is an expression
      of conscious opposition, request that Centrum reveal that
      information to consciousness.

      Centrum, please elevate to consciousness the memories of
      those experiences in which you learned to experience asthma,
      as well as understanding of the work you just completed.
      Please do so by writing on the chalkboard, by an inner
      voice, memory, insight or any other means. Please write the C – 115
      word "complete" when you have done so.   F – 214

115   Inquire if the patient is satisfied with the information
      received. Ask if it all makes sense and if the patient could,
      if requested, describe the process by which the asthma
      became a part of his life. If satisfied, go to Step 116. If not
      satisfied, go back to Step 114 and persuade Centrum to
      reveal the information, or determine if one or more parts
      are preventing conscious awareness. In the latter case, guide

Centrum to communicate with those parts, persuading them   S – 116
to permit conscious awareness.   N – 114

116 Express to the patient the fact that the real test of
completeness of this work is in the real world, yet there is
value in finding a way to test it here and now, so that if not
complete, we can continue the process now. Ask the patient
to use his or her imagination to project into the future, into
a situation in which an asthma attack would be expected to
occur. If the patient has difficulty imagining that situation,
the work is not complete and Centrum should be asked to
identify the part. Other tests may occur to you. Use them as   F – 216
necessary as an aid in decisions of the moment.   S – 117

117 The task of change is now complete insofar as it is possible
to test at this point. Explain to the patient that, although it
appears to be complete, the real test is in the real world, and
that some additional part might have escaped detection and
still be active causing the asthma. Assure the patient that if
there is a continuation of the asthma, it simply means that
the work is not yet complete and that taking succeeding
steps will be even more efficiently accomplished, now that
Centrum knows how to do the work more efficiently. To not
provide the assurance that the work can be finally completed
– even if the asthma should recur – is to risk premature
withdrawal from treatment. Point out that recurrence would
simply mean the work is not complete; it does not mean
failure of the person or of the treatment.

Excellent work, Centrum. Thank you.

200 SERIES

200 It may seem incongruous that Centrum is not aware of what
is happening in the patient's life, yet that sometimes occurs,
and the patient is usually dysfunctional because of it. Your
task is to make Centrum aware of the issue and one way
is to ask the patient to verbalize the problem, in simple yet
comprehensive terms, after requesting that Centrum listen.   100

201 At this point in the process, you are dependent
upon Centrum. It is necessary that Centrum develop
understanding of causal factors and it is your job to
facilitate this. It might be that Centrum simply does not
understand what is expected, or that Centrum is unable
to overcome the blocking of some resistant part, or other
issue. By appropriate questions to Centrum, based on your
professional sense of the situation, clarify the problem and
persuade Centrum to continue with the work.   101

202   Your request may not be clear for a number of reasons; however, it is probably due to your not having phrased the request in terms Centrum could follow. Rephrase it as required, perhaps including a review of the concepts of Subliminal Therapy, and repeat the question.

Centrum, please investigate this issue. Review memories of events that may have had something to do with it and communicate with those parts that are involved. The objective, Centrum, is for you to understand how asthma became part of your life. Centrum, is my request clear to you?

Y – 103
N – 202

203   If you have requested that Centrum indicate when the task is complete by writing "complete" on the chalkboard, and there has been no response, it may be that you (or the patient) are being impatient and Centrum simply needs more time. Ask Centrum if that is the case.

Centrum, are you involved in the process and need more time? If the answer is "Yes": Okay, we will be patient, just let us know by the word "complete" when you have completed the task.

C – 104

204   Rephrase your request to Centrum. You must depend upon Centrum's ability to access memories etc., and perhaps Centrum did not understand your request as you intended it. Ensure that you speak of Centrum using the abilities of memory access, communication with other parts, etc., to uncover the needed information.

104

205   It is possible that Centrum is actively causing the problem that is the focus of treatment. Centrum may disagree with the conscious opinion of the patient.

Centrum, are you, Centrum, are you causing [problem]?

N – 105
Y – 302

206   Repeat your request using different words and include elaboration and explanation as you sense is necessary.

106

207   Although usually not a problem, this question may not be understood by Centrum. Explain that it will be necessary for Centrum to communicate with the identified parts and that this step is necessary to set the stage for that to happen.

107

208   You may, or you may not, know how many parts are actually involved causing the presenting problem; you only know there are more than one. Ask Centrum to select one of the parts and to proceed with the protocol. When Centrum has

cleared that part, ask Centrum to select another, and then
another, until all have been cleared.   109

209   Your task is that of establishing communication between
Centrum and the identified part. While the part may not be
willing to communicate, it is usually willing to consider new
information if doing so does not require self-disclosure.

Centrum, are you willing to communicate with the part?   Y – 303
                                                            N – 310

210   Somehow there has been a lack of clear communication to
Centrum. Perhaps it had to do with phrasing, or even with
content. Repeat the instructions of Step 110 in different
words, checking incrementally with Centrum to ensure
understanding.   110

211   You have requested that Centrum indicate completeness
by writing the word "complete" and no response has been
forthcoming. Ask Centrum if more time is needed. If no, ask
if Centrum is willing to do the work.

Centrum, are you willing to establish communication and   Y – 111
do the work as requested?   N – 101

212   *Centrum, did you succeed in establishing communication*   Y – 110
with the part, as I requested?   N – 209

214   Unconscious entities may deny conscious awareness for
reasons of protection or for other reasons that are considered
valid. On the other hand, it may be that conscious awareness
is not necessary to accomplish the goal. You won't know
unless you ask.

Centrum, will conscious awareness be necessary to   Y – 114
accomplish the goal?   N – 308

216   Inability to imagine the desired situation without difficulty is
clear indication that the work is not complete.

Centrum, the work is apparently not complete. I therefore
ask that you reinvestigate the beginning of the asthma and
learn what remains to be accomplished. Identify the part(s)
that continue to be active in causing the asthma.   C – 104

300 SERIES

302 You need to know Centrum's reason for causing the asthma, since this is the root of the barrier to the consciously desired change. So ask Centrum to write that reason, or to express by an inner voice, or by other means. When the reason is expressed, guide the patient to offer countering views – back and forth – until agreement is reached, then proceed on that agreement.

303 In this step, you are seeking a way to engineer communication between the part and Centrum. A fair assumption is that the part is fearful of exposure and the following approach has been highly effective in resolving the barrier.

Centrum, is the part willing to consider information with the provision that it need not expose itself, that it is only required to listen?

Y – 305
N – 304

A "no" response to this question will challenge your professional ability to devise an approach that will overcome the barrier. One possible approach is to temporarily abandon Subliminal Therapy, perhaps using age-regression techniques to resolve the immediate aspect, then return to working with Subliminal Therapy. Perhaps request Centrum to select a different part to work with, then come back to this part after requesting the part to listen to the process.

304 *Centrum, please communicate with the part. Inform the part about present life conditions, needs, values and desires. Ensure that the part understands the negative consequences of its influence and persuade the part to support your conscious goals.*

305 Here, the best bet is to assume that the part is, in fact, listening and to ask Centrum to communicate as though that is true. Assume the part is well-intended and appeal to that good intention

Centrum, please communicate information to this part, information about present life conditions etc. Be supportive of that part, Centrum, appeal to its good intentions.

C – 110

306 The part agreed to listen, and apparently has listened to the appeal from Centrum. The next step is to engineer bilateral communications between the part and Centrum so that full, mutual understanding can be reached between them.

> *Centrum, is the part now willing to communicate fully with*   Y – 304
> *you in an exchange of positions and opinions?*   N – 110

307   *Centrum, please communicate further information to the*
part. This time, Centrum, appeal to the positive intention of
the part, offer any information you believe may persuade the
part to communicate with you.   C – 110

308   Make it clear that you are asking for the conscious opinion
of the patient, ask if it is important to him or her to know, at
a conscious level, about the work just completed. Some will
insist on knowing, others will not want to know.

> *[Patient's name], do you want to know, to understand*   Y – 309
> *consciously, what Centrum just accomplished?*   N – 408

309   The patient wants to know, and there is value in having
that knowledge, therefore, this becomes the focus of
therapy. With this goal in mind, guide Centrum to eliminate
the barrier, perhaps by following the basic protocol of
Subliminal Therapy.

310   There are many conceivable reasons why Centrum might be
unwilling to continue. You might be able to anticipate the
reason and respond effectively, or you might not know the
reason. Ask if Centrum is willing to reveal the reason for
the refusal and use this response (if provided) to persuade
Centrum.

Your talents as a clinician will be tested at this juncture. Be
inventive, knowing that unless Centrum can be persuaded,
you must shift to another mode of treatment.

400 SERIES

408   In some instances, patients are just curious about what
is going on, in other cases they may strongly desire to
know, and in other cases they may not want to know. As
the clinician, you are obligated to conform to the patient's
wishes insofar as you are able to do so; after all, it is the
patient's life. It might be that the prospect of knowing what
actually happened is so overwhelming that the patient is
unwilling to continue therapy; it is seen as a threat that must
not be accommodated. Pay attention to your instincts.

Appendix B

General Information to be Provided to the Patient before Treatment

The following brief essays have served me well in informing and guiding my patients down an effective, therapeutic path. They present issues that have typically arisen in the course of treating patients over the years and are included in my ST booklet for patients (Yager, 1985). If I have prior knowledge of the presenting problem, I will ensure that the patient is exposed to the pertinent essay during the initial procedure. If new issues become apparent in the course of treatment, I will introduce additional content at that point. The information is provided for the patient to consider, not as statements of absolute reality or values.

Smooth Muscle

To understand the mechanism whereby psychological conditioning affects the physical body, it is necessary to consider the function of smooth muscle.

The musculature of the human body is divided into three classes: skeletal, smooth and cardiac. Skeletal muscles are those muscles we employ to move the limbs of our body, to walk, talk and lift things. We consciously control skeletal muscles. Examples of smooth muscles include those muscles that propel food through the digestive system, that control the pattern of blood flow in the body by variably occluding the arteries and those involved with respiration. Moreover, the glands themselves consist of smooth muscles which act in concert with ducts. Cardiac muscles are the muscles of the heart – the muscles that pump blood through the circulatory system.

Smooth and cardiac muscles are controlled by unconscious functioning of the mind; with few exceptions, they are not subject to conscious, volitional control. Under unconscious control, they actuate the processes that maintain life, doing so in a manner so sophisticated that it is beyond our conscious ability even to comprehend. The essential factor to be understood in all of this is that, aside from conscious control of skeletal muscles, the action of smooth muscles is the link between mental and physical interactions. When the mind is at peace, the body is at peace, functioning as it should. When the mind is disturbed, the body becomes disturbed by the action of smooth muscles outside of conscious control.

Many physical disorders are directly caused by the action of smooth muscle. Bronchial asthma, for example, is a potentially life-threatening illness that occurs when smooth muscles occlude the air passageways in the lungs and throat. Irritable bowel syndrome is the consequence of smooth muscles in the stomach, coupled with the action of related glands, disrupting the digestive process. Tension and migraine headaches are caused by smooth muscles creating cranial pressure. The etiology of these disorders may thus be psychogenic and, in my experience, commonly are.

Since the action of smooth muscle is controlled unconsciously, it makes sense to treat psychogenic illness by correcting the unconscious processes causing the problem, and ST is the intervention of choice. By its use, the unconscious causes of the illness can be uncovered and resolved; the symptoms then cease to exist.

Emotions

Four emotions – fear, guilt, bitterness and grief – form the roots of most human unhappiness. The following essays provide food for thought about these emotions for consideration.

Fear

Fear is a universal human experience that is absolutely necessary for survival. Without fear, we would do things that would result in injury or death. However, sometimes the fear we experience is not necessary and results in undesirable experiences or dysfunctions.

Innate vs. learned fears. A few fears seem truly innate. An infant will react in ways that indicate fear in response to a sudden noise and to being dropped an inch or so. More common fears, however, are learned. A small child will not hesitate to touch something hot, to put dangerous things in his mouth or to approach a threatening animal. The child must learn to avoid these things, that is, he must learn to respond with fear in their presence.

We may fear the unknown, the most common of fears, even though it is seldom based in reality. Fears may be learned, and may even be products of our imagination, having no basis in reality. Of course, it occasionally turns out that there is some real basis for a fear. Yet even then, when the basis becomes known, we are usually able to cope with the situation.

Rational vs. irrational fears. Some of the fears we learn are wholly rational, as in the cases mentioned above. However, sometimes we learn to fear in an irrational or distorted way, and these fears may take place without conscious awareness of their cause. For example, a child, frightened in a dark place may learn to fear the dark, and that learned fear may persist for a lifetime. The child is not aware that he is learning to fear the dark, and while it is entirely rational that he would do so in that situation, it is irrational for him, as an adult, to continue to do so.

Conscious vs. unconscious fears. To further understand fear, we must consider the possibility that it may be experienced at an unconscious level of awareness, with only its effect being experienced consciously. Fear of the unknown may simply be fear of something known at an unconscious level, yet not known consciously. An example might be a fear of people of another race, or a fear reaction to a sound or situation, without the reasons being known consciously. In other words, we may have learned to fear something at some time in the past and not have conscious memory of having done so.

The concept of experiencing fear unconsciously may seem unusual. Yet a moment's reflection provides several illustrations of this happening: the unconscious may protect us by keeping us 'big', thus armoring us against being hurt by producing a weight problem; the unconscious may keep us in a state of readiness for fight-or-flight, resulting in various gastro-intestinal disorders such as colitis or ulcers; or the unconscious may cause us to be introverted rather than to risk criticism.

On the other hand, we may have conscious awareness of the thing that is feared without awareness of why it is feared or of the reason for its intensity, as in the case of a phobia. It is also possible we may have neither conscious nor unconscious awareness of the thing that is feared or of why it is feared. Beyond that, we may have no conscious experience of fear at all, even though the unconscious may respond by producing protective reactions in the form of behaviors or dysfunctions which consciously appear irrational.

Unconscious parts of the mind often control behavior in response to influences that were learned in past situations, that is, at the time the parts came into existence. Such behavior can be understood best when considered in the light of the limited knowledge that was available at that time. For example, the limited knowledge of the small child might result in the child approaching and being attacked by an animal with a consequent phobia of that animal.

The effects of fear. The effects of fear may be either physical, psychological or a combination of both, and may range from minor nuisance to severe illness. One psychological result is a phobia. Another might be hostility that manifests itself in obvious or subtle ways. A frightened, cornered animal will exhibit hostility that is the product of fear, the fear being basically a protective device.

Whether conscious or unconscious, a prolonged experience of fear will usually result in some physical dysfunction which may be recognized as illness. And such dysfunction may become evident in any organ or portion of the body. Many physical changes take place when we experience fear, changes that affect virtually every organ of our bodies. These changes are geared to provide the inner physical conditions needed for fight-or-flight. Examples: When fear is experienced, the pattern of blood flow in the body changes so that the muscle systems involved in physical action are amply supplied at the expense of less essential functions such as digestion, which may cease altogether; glandular activity which is dramatically altered with consequent change in muscle tone; breathing patterns which are altered; and in the reduction of time required for blood coagulation. Most such changes that take place would be regarded as illness if reported in the absence of consciously experienced fear. In summary, many physical ailments may have their genesis in conflicts or fears of which we are consciously unaware.

The resolution of fears. We may learn to fear things that are known to be the cause of our reaction, or we may learn to fear the unknown. When these things are known, we are generally able to cope with them by rational means; we may talk ourselves out of it, or make use of its energy in some productive way. Or we may obtain relief simply by considering its basis in a rational way, reframing our understanding.

In resolving an irrational fear, it may be helpful to consider probabilities. We know logically that almost anything we can conceive of is possible, and that to completely avoid danger we would have to stay in bed. And yet, we couldn't safely stay in bed either, because some danger exists even then, such as earthquakes, fires, cyclones, etc. We cannot continue to exist without some degree of risk. We know that is true, and we are able to function in spite of that knowledge, because we also know that it is highly probable that no harm will befall us. Rational consideration of the situation, perhaps just stopping to think about it a moment, will often put things in the perspective of reality, thereby resolving the fear.

However, when we fear the unknown, we are prevented from consciously confronting its cause, and we must rely on our unconscious abilities to resolve that fear. After all, it is an unconscious problem and it will require an unconscious solution. Guided by your therapist, and relying on your unconscious abilities, a solution can usually be found.

Guilt

In its most basic form, guilt is the consequence of a decision: a decision to do or not to do, something that one now feels guilty about. That decision may have been made after reasoned consideration, or it may have been made – as many decisions are made – in response to emotional influence without appropriate, rational consideration. Even in spite of rational consideration, our (learned) values impose a great many 'shoulds' and 'shouldn'ts' on our behavior. And while the values we hold can largely be traced to parental teachings, any source we considered authoritative may have contributed. If we behave contrary to values we learned as a child we may feel guilt, even if we no longer hold the particular value to be valid. Then too, guilt may be unconsciously experienced, manifesting in various ways and requiring intervention at the unconscious level for elimination.

Decisions as a source of guilt. We make a great many decisions in life, hundreds of them every day. Most have no serious consequence, for example, whether first to take out the trash or feed the dog, but occasionally a decision of real importance comes along and, much more rarely, we must make a decision having real life impact. However, *all* of these decisions, from the least significant to the most important, have three elements in common:

- *All* decisions are made without enough information. 'Enough' information would at least require knowledge about consequence, and such knowledge is not available at the time of decision.

- *All* decisions are influenced by emotions, and sometimes we make decisions wholly for emotional reasons, even against rational judgment. We are often unable even to distinguish between emotional reaction and rational process, and we may rationalize emotional reasons, thereby disguising them.

- *All* decisions are influenced by things outside of ourselves, e.g., the situation, someone else's needs and/or any number of other possible factors.

If we accept the premise that every decision is made on the basis of the above three factors, a fundamental lesson emerges: If those factors are the *only* factors involved, then it appears the decision made was the only decision that could have been made! For another decision to have been made would have required that at least one of the three factors be different than it was.

As an aid to understanding this concept, consider some decision you have made in light of the above three factors:

- Was it possible for you to have known more than you knew? Was it possible for you to change your values about the issues involved?

- Was it possible for you to change the emotional experience of the moment? Likely, it was no more possible than it is possible for you to arbitrarily change what you are experiencing at this moment.

- Was it possible for you to change outside reality? What was there was there. You could neither have added to, nor subtracted from, that reality.

Given these truths, it becomes apparent that you made the only decision it was possible for you to have made.

The understanding that the decision made was the only decision that could have been made permits self-forgiveness and, through forgiving, a release from guilt. In any event, you may be aware that the decision you made was the best decision you could have made given those factors as they were, even though the decision may now be viewed as a mistake.

Values as a source of guilt. Sometimes we are made to feel guilty by the imposition of someone else's values. This happens all too often with children and well-intentioned parents. Of course it is necessary and desirable to teach the child the values of the parents; this is the way of life. On the other hand, it is neither necessary nor desirable that values be taught by making the child feel guilty for some act, or for some mistake made. The time-honored admonition, "Punish the act and praise the child" can be employed as a cardinal rule for parents to teach values without imposing guilt.

Even after childhood, our values change as we learn more about ourselves and the world in which we live. If we violate a value today, and feel guilt and remorse for doing so, what about tomorrow if we no longer hold that value to be valid? What about the guilt that was so real yesterday? And, what about the effect of the guilt that may persist? Children sometimes assume blame, with consequent guilt, for events that take place. And, even though the child may later understand that the blame was misplaced, such guilt can have serious consequences of lifelong duration. This can be especially true if the event is consciously forgotten, leaving the guilt to be experienced unconsciously.

Unconscious guilt. Any emotion, most certainly including guilt, can be experienced by the unconscious mind without conscious awareness. Moreover, we may have conscious awareness of the effect of an unconscious emotion without conscious awareness of its cause. The most frequent effect of unconscious guilt is a compulsion for self-punishment, the results of which may be quite obvious indeed. We may behave in ways that preclude success. We may overeat or physically abuse ourselves in other ways. We may not be able to experience joy, even though we observe the experience in others. These and a great many other possible ways of punishing ourselves may be unconsciously devised and enforced without our being consciously aware of why. Other possible means of self-punishment include obesity, self-mutilation, psychogenic illness and suicide.

Utilizing guilt. Some people believe that guilt is a necessary and desirable experience, that its influence is effective in controlling behavior. They hold that without guilt human behavior would be intolerable. To the extent that we are able to learn by feeling guilt, that position would seem valid. However, behavioral psychology has convincingly shown that reward, not punishment, is the preferred way to modify behavior, and guilt is another form of punishment. It therefore seems that the value of guilt in regulating behavior is at least questionable, and is likely outweighed by probable negative consequences.

Another equally ill-advised use of guilt is its use as a defensive measure. A person who has done something he considers wrong may use guilt as evidence that he is really okay. "After all," he might say, "I did it, but at least I feel bad (guilty) about it." In this sense, he is compensating for what he did by feeling guilty. To release the guilt would restore the intolerable state of mind that prompted the guilt to begin with. Freedom from that state of mind more than compensates for any consequence of the guilt itself. For such a person, eliminating guilt will require a different way of looking at what happened and at the consequences of the guilt that ensued.

Resolution of guilt. Forgiving one's self through understanding is the way to resolve guilt. You must seek new information that provides new understanding. Unconscious memory contains a storehouse of information about the self. It seems literally true that we never forget anything! Everything we ever perceived made an impression, a recording of some sort. We may not have access to all memories at our conscious will and pleasure, but they are there, and we can have access to at least some of them under the right circumstances. By reviewing those memories, we can gain understanding of the factors that produced guilt. And by understanding those factors in the light of present knowledge, we may recognize that the guilt is misplaced or inappropriate. This new understanding may be accomplished at a conscious level of awareness, or it may be accomplished at an unconscious level, without conscious awareness. As you employ the technique of Subliminal Therapy, learning to depend upon your unconscious abilities, you may consciously experience benefits without necessarily understanding their origin. Release from guilt is but one such benefit.

Bitterness

To be bitter is to be unhappy. To experience bitterness is to occupy one's mind with imagery and feelings of repressed anger that prevent pleasurable experiences and productive thought.

To be bitter is to experience energy which is almost certainly exerted in the wrong direction, energy that does not affect the object of the bitterness, yet may be devastating to the one who is bitter.

Bitterness is usually the consequence of taking personal offense to something someone has done or has not done. If the personal element of the offense is taken away, only disagreement remains, and disagreement need not be destructive.

Bitterness is usually experienced toward someone who is, or has been, close to you. The same injustice committed by a stranger would not have the same personal impact. Taking things personally means you assume that the act in question was done deliberately to affect *you*, to hurt *you*. Truthfully, the *real* reason for the act had nothing whatever to do with you. It had only to do with the other person's values, beliefs, motivations and behavior – all products of that person's life conditioning.

We are all products of conditioning, and the things we do are products of that conditioning too, not just products of the present situation. We may respond with anger to a situation in which another would respond with humor. How we respond depends upon how we have learned to respond, and this is also true of that other person. No matter what the hurtful act was, it resulted from the other person's conditioning; we could only have functioned as the stimulus.

To clarify this concept, consider the example of a child who is physically abused by a parent. The child perceives the abuse in a personal way and the psychological damage that results, the guilt or the dissociation, is a consequence of that perspective. Much less damage would result if the child were capable of perceiving that the *real* reason for the abuse had nothing whatever to do with them; the real reason for the abuse was there before the child was even conceived. In like manner, the *real* reason for the act about which you are bitter had nothing to do with you.

The key to releasing one's self from bitterness is to forgive. And to forgive requires not will power, but understanding. If by meditation, discussion or reasoning, you are able to gain insight into the motivation of the offending other, you will release some portion of bitterness. And even if information about the other's motivation is not available, understanding that it has nothing to do with you personally will afford release. Forgiving is for your own benefit, not for the benefit of the other, although the other may also benefit.

Grief

It is universally human to grieve. We may grieve over the loss of a loved one, the loss of an animal, the loss of a job, the loss of our youth or the loss of some material object. However, in all events, grief involves loss, and loss is an unavoidable part of life. In grief, the mind is monopolized by awareness of loss to such an extent that the normal view of life becomes distorted. We may become incapable of reasoned judgment and rational decision.

Working through grief. Working through grief is a process of re-establishing appropriate and realistic perspective about our values, and of re-establishing the ability to reason. In essence, it is a process of transferring mental activity from an awareness of loss in the past to an awareness of present reality, including strengths, abilities and assets.

Working through grief is not just a conscious activity; it involves unconscious reorganization as well. When we grieve, it is as though a newly created part of the unconscious mind – the part aware of loss – dominates the other parts in the same way that an angry, fearful or guilty part may dominate in other situations. Working through grief becomes a process of education in which the grieving parts of the mind become aware of values and reality as understood consciously. Working through grief can involve a developing awareness of the beginning of a new life, a life with new needs, new responsibilities and new problems to be addressed that are different from the needs, responsibilities and problems as they were before.

The steps described in following paragraphs have proven effective as an organized, structured way of working through grief. Deliberate, conscious consideration of these steps appears to make the necessary unconscious work possible. Although the reality of the loss is unchanged, the perception of that reality is changed, and the grief may thereby be resolved.

First, it seems important to identify and acknowledge whatever emotions are present now, in the present moment, doing so by means of words, not just vague impressions. If you are grieving, take these steps: First, identify the emotions you are experiencing by name. You may feel sadness, anger, fear or other emotions. Acknowledge whatever is there by calm introspection.

Second, identify the needs which had been satisfied by the lost relationship. Some will be obvious, some much less so. Reliance on the unconscious for communicating awareness and understanding to consciousness is important here. Pay attention to spontaneous thoughts and insights as they are apt to be communications from your unconscious mind. Defining needs makes it possible to consider the means by which those needs may be satisfied in the future.

The third step involves thinking through new responsibilities, to self as well as to others, that apply to your new life. Each responsibility must be recognized before steps can be taken to meet them, and once recognized the steps necessary often become apparent.

The fourth step is to define the problems presented by this new life situation, and then to consider possible solutions to those problems. Again, depend upon your unconscious abilities, paying attention to communications from your unconscious mind. The recognition that multiple, possible solutions exist is reassuring and often dispels feelings of helplessness.

The final step is to permit awareness that ongoing positive influence from the lost relationship endures. The lessons learned and the strengths developed in the course of that relationship are valuable and persist into your present and your future. Again, be introspective. Be curious about what thoughts and insights may occur to you.

Experience

The concepts of selfishness, forgiving and acceptance presented here are offered to stimulate your thinking, and perhaps to present a different way of thinking about them.

Selfishness

Most of us were taught that it is wrong to be selfish. That lesson is impressed upon us in many ways by parents, school and church. However, there is another way of thinking about selfishness. Perhaps selfishness is neither wrong nor right; perhaps it is simply a fact of life, a fact that has not been clearly understood. With but a little thought, most would agree that we are selfish beings; it is the way we were created. If that view is accurate, then either selfishness is good or we are fundamentally bad. Conversely, since we are apparently not fundamentally bad, selfishness must be good. It is good because it provides us with the motivation to do good things, things we would not do at all were we not selfishly motivated to do them. We *must* do things to satisfy our own needs, and many things we do for ourselves benefit others as well. In this view, selfishness is seen as a virtue.

When we act unselfishly, or make a decision for unselfish reasons, there are apt to be negative consequences. One typical consequence is guilt; another is bitterness. A child may be told,

"You should want to share your toy." And while the child may be required to share the toy, the child cannot be made to *want* to do so. The child may, however, be made to feel guilty for not wanting to share, and in this event an injury is done. It is natural for the child to be selfish. An adult required to share a valued possession would feel the same.

We often do things for the benefit of others, and when we do, we do so for selfish reasons. We are rewarded by the good feelings we get from the act, by the pleasure we take in pleasing someone or by the reflection of love or appreciation shown by that other person. If we benefit from the act, if we derive pleasure or profit in some way, then we are motivated to act. This is the positive side of selfishness, and without its influence we would do nothing at all. When we express love, we do so because we are motivated to do so. When we give away a possession, we do so because we are motivated to so do. And the root of such motivation is selfishness.

When we marry, we marry for selfish reasons; no marriage could be happy otherwise. Can you imagine marrying against your will? We must be honestly selfish in that situation for our own benefit as well as for the benefit of the person we marry. In the same manner, we tend to be selfish in every decision we make. To do otherwise, to make a decision for someone else's sake, against our own wishes, is to invite resentment. And resentment affects all others with whom we are in contact.

To further illustrate these principles, consider the example of a parent who is unhappy in a marriage, a parent who urgently and sincerely wants to be free of the marriage, and yet who for the sake of the children stays in the marriage. The consequences of such an unselfish decision will almost certainly be resentment, if not overt bitterness. Not even the children, for whom the sacrifice was made, are protected from that consequence.

Consider these viewpoints about selfishness:

- Being selfish is not just okay, it is essential to our happiness. And if we are unhappy, we influence others to be unhappy.

And if we are happy, we influence others to be happy. We must be selfish if we are to satisfy our own needs, and if we neglect our own needs, we are weakened and so are less able to be of value to others.

- Being selfish does not mean that we should steal, lie or cheat; the contrary is true. By doing such things, we demean our-selves in our own image, a guaranteed path to unhappiness. And so, for very selfish reasons, we should not to do such things.

- An advantage of sharing unselfishly is that others are encouraged to share in return and we thus expand our expe-riences. In helping another, we enhance our self-image and so benefit in many subtle ways. It is therefore in our selfish interest to share.

- In making ourselves desirable – to spouse or to friend – we benefit from the attention returned, just as they benefit from our attention to them. The Biblical Golden Rule, "Do unto others as you would have them do unto you," is a selfishly advisable rule.

We are often made to feel guilty for being selfish by parents, friends, teachers and critics. Recognition that selfishness is a real-ity of life, experienced by those very parents, friends, teachers and critics, provides relief from the guilt that is imposed by such sources. It is truly okay for you to be you, and for me to be me, and that includes being selfish. It is okay for us to benefit from the motivation and from the productive direction in life that self-ishness provides. It is okay because we, and all those influenced by us, benefit from it.

Forgiveness

If we blame ourselves for something, we may experience guilt. If we blame another, we may experience bitterness. Either way, we lose. Guilt and bitterness are sources of a great deal of unhap-piness. To experience either is to use mental energy in negative ways that prolong those feelings by excluding productive thought and by distorting reality. Forgiving, either one's self or others, is the way out of the traps of guilt and bitterness.

We are taught that it is good to forgive, yet we are seldom taught how to forgive. The implication is that forgiving is an act of will. Forgiveness, however, seems not to be a matter of will; forgiving seems possible only through a change in understanding. Forgiveness is not an act; it is not something we do. Forgiveness is something we *experience* when we achieve new understanding that changes our perspective.

When we consider the 'facts' from a different perspective, our understanding may change, and with a changed understanding, we feel differently about whatever happened. These two thoughts about guilt make sense:

- Whatever you did – or did not do – that you feel guilty about was the consequence of the way you had been conditioned to behave up to that point in time.

- Given the same situation and the same influences again, you'd respond the same way again. You would do – or not do – what you did the first time.

Consider the experience of bitterness. Bitterness is a source of much energy, every bit of which is exerted in the wrong direction. Bitterness can truly destroy, but the destruction takes place within the one who is bitter, not in the one toward whom the bitterness is directed. Test this concept by applying it to your own life. You will find ample reason to forgive, and forgiving is a matter of considering the reasons for the bitterness from another perspective.

Bitterness ceases to exist when we forgive. It is important to recognize that the other person is caught in the same web of conditioning that we are caught in. That other person is doing precisely what he or she has been conditioned to do. After all, if he had been conditioned differently, he would have behaved differently. By giving that person room to do what he is going to do anyway, we cease to judge him by our values. And the moment we do that, the moment we permit that person to function according to values other than our own, we experience forgiveness. And we also experience the benefits that forgiveness provides *us*.

It is indeed good to forgive. It is in our selfish interest to forgive. There is a release of negative energy that can profoundly improve our lives. To be sure, another may benefit indirectly, but the real benefit is enjoyed by the one who forgives. That is the person relieved of a burden, a burden that is guaranteed to prevent happiness.

Another important consideration is that blame is nonsensical; it is irrational and has no place in a reasoned scheme of life. Blaming ourselves produces guilt; blaming another person produces resentment. Forgiving eliminates blame – as well as the guilt and resentment.

Consider yet another illustration of the principles of forgiving. A child who is abused by a parent is abused for reasons that have nothing to do with the child; the reasons for the abuse were there long before the child was even conceived. The adult who is persecuted because of race is persecuted for reasons that have nothing whatever to do with that person as a person; the reasons have only to do with the conditioning of the persecutor. This is not to defend abuse or persecution, as these are wrong by any intelligent standard of values. Rather, this is an attempt to explain their existence, thereby creating opportunity for the abused to escape the injury that persists. Remember that new understanding can make forgiving possible.

If someone criticizes us, we often react defensively. Such is our nature. And as long as we are defending the way we are (or what we did), we are stuck as we are; we are unable to change, even though we may wish to do so. When we forgive, we cease to be critical and, freed from the need to defend, change becomes possible. Incidentally, that becomes a good test of forgiving; if we are still critical, we have not forgiven.

Just as forgiveness eliminates criticism, it also eliminates the need to be defensive. It thereby encourages new perspective and change.

In summary, to forgive does *not* require acceptance or approval of the offending behavior, either on the part of another or of ourselves. Forgiving may, however, make change possible if that change is desired. In the final analysis, forgiving is a wholly selfish process, and it is selfishness that provides the motivation to forgive. It is only incidental that another may benefit.

Acceptance

We believe what we were conditioned to believe. We do what we were conditioned to do. And we were not consulted about how we wanted to have been conditioned. The result is that we hold opinions and display attitudes and behaviors that are quite beyond our ability to change, even though we may wish to do so. Fortunately, at least on the surface, we usually seem able to accept ourselves as we are, and we may staunchly defend the way we are and our right to be that way. At the same time, we may be critical of someone else for being as he is. In some situations, we may want (and even expect) the other person to change, to conform to our values or to satisfy our needs. We may also be surprised and severely disappointed when the change we want is not forthcoming. The concept of acceptance, as I present it, may help you avoid that surprise and disappointment.

We encounter many situations in life in which the behavior of a person who is important to us can cause us to react in an undesirable way. If we are married to that person, or committed, or involved in any binding way, the consequence can be frustrating for all concerned and can effectively eliminate harmony from the relationship. Acceptance, as presented here, is a means of interacting, of relating with another in harmony.

Acceptance is a selfish act. As a means of restoring harmony to a stressed relationship, you may consider accepting that other person as is, without expecting that they be different in any way. You may want to accept the other, but in a special way. Acceptance, in the sense used here, does not mean that you have to agree with the other person. Accepting does not mean that you must like or approve of what they do. Accepting means simply that you recognize and acknowledge that the other person is doing precisely what they have been conditioned to do. Then, with that recognition, you are able to give them room to do, and be, what they are going to do and be anyway, whether or not you give room, without your expressing or even feeling criticism.

Consider what would be required for *you* to change an opinion you hold about something. You might change that opinion if you were to learn something new. However, it is not possible to simply and arbitrarily change your opinion without new information of some kind. That other person is in exactly the same position, and your dismay that he does not agree with you is communicated to him as criticism or rejection.

You may be reacting negatively to what another is doing (or is not doing) that you think should (or should not) be done. Consider what would be required for *you* to do something differently, for you to stop reacting the way you are reacting at this moment. It is obviously not within your power to arbitrarily change your reaction, and neither is it within the power of the other to change, arbitrarily, to conform to your values.

It is obviously possible to demand that another do as you might wish. You can enforce your demand with a gun, with psychological pressure, with threat of leaving or with other means of coercion. However, by doing so you have not changed the values the other holds and the result is always resentment. Even though the resentment may not be overtly expressed (and perhaps not even recognized consciously), it does gain expression in covert ways that can be destructive to all concerned.

Consider a situation in which the wife – for whatever reasons she may have – does not keep the house as clean as her husband – for whatever reasons he may have – believes she should. Assuming that the feelings are intense, and that there is significant threat to the relationship because of those feelings and that neither wants the relationship to end. What now? The surface issue is that of a clean house; the underlying issue is that the husband is dissatisfied with things as they are, and the wife is satisfied with things as they are. The problem, in other words, is apparently his, not hers. He is demanding change, not she. Therefore, he must seek a solution, or it is unlikely that a solution will be found. Since he cannot force her to change (he has been trying that for years), he must solve his problem outside of her. He can clean the house himself or pay someone else to do it. He can fake a change in his own values in a way that makes the house okay as it is, or do nothing at all and live with his frustration. Or he can solve his problem by divorce. Obviously none of these solutions is really satisfactory, since none of them resolves the relationship problem; no matter which solution he chooses, resentment and consequent rejection ensues.

This problem is a common one and involves a variety of issues besides a clean house. The solution of such problems seems possible only by a change in perspective on the part of the one demanding change, since they are the only one motivated to bring the change about. The most productive step possible in the preceding example would be that of his accepting her. Then it wouldn't matter which of the clean house solutions he chooses to employ. If he is truly able to embrace, *as reality*, the fact that she is as she is, thereby making it okay for her to be as she is, he can clean the house (or pay to have it done) without feeling resentment. Or he can re-examine his own values without feeling forced to do so, or take whatever other steps seem best, doing so in good grace, rewarded by the peace and harmony in the relationship that his acceptance of her produces.

To further illustrate the principles involved in accepting, suppose that: (1) you are married to someone; (2) you wish to continue to be married to that person; (3) you are unhappy because of some habit or characteristic of that person; (4) despite all pleading, threatening, cajoling and pressuring, the person has not changed as you would like; (5) you are not willing for the situation to continue as it is; (6) the situation is continuing as it is; and (7) you wish to continue to be married to that person and … If you are experiencing something like this, you are locked into a cause/effect cycle that can endure for a lifetime. And it *is* within your power to interrupt that cycle. You can do so by simply accepting your spouse, by allowing him or her to do, be and say what he or she is going to do, be and say anyway, no matter how dumb, wrong or objectionable you may think it to be. Remember, you do not have to agree or approve of what the other is doing. You need only accept the person, not the person's behavior. You might say something like, "I don't like what you are doing but I accept that you have to do it for some reason, so I'll get off your back about it." Or you might say: "You're really convinced about that aren't you? I don't agree, but I accept that you really believe it." Or "That hurt me! It hurt especially because you are so important to me! And I want you to know that it hurt me!"

When you respond to another in a way that is different from the way you usually respond, the other must respond differently to us. If you have always responded to an attack with an attack in return, your adversary will be surprised and off balance if you respond with acceptance of their position, attitude or belief. If you respond to a criticism with an awareness of the other's position, rather than with a criticism in return, then the other *must* respond to you in a different way. The good news is: that different way is likely to be non-aggressive and may even be supportive of you!

The key to responding differently is to accept the other, to accept the reality that the other holds a different viewpoint and to allow that viewpoint to exist as the sincere expression that it is. The adage about raising children, "Punish the act and praise the child" works for adults as well. Separate the person from what the person is doing. Accept the person and it is okay to reject what the person does.

As long as you struggle to require change in someone else, you are denying that person's individuality. You may not know the reason why someone believes or behaves as they do, and they probably do not know why themselves; however, you know some things about that reason. You know that it exists, because if it did not exist, or if it were different, the person would behave or believe differently. You also know that the reason is a product of that person's conditioning and almost certainly has nothing whatever to do with you! Whatever the reason, it was there before you were there and so is actually not a reflection on you. It has nothing to do with you personally. It has only to do with the other's conditioning, with things that happened before you came into the picture. As I expressed before, a child abused by a parent is abused for reasons that have nothing to do with the child.

Acceptance eliminates controversy. By accepting your spouse (or friend, boss, or …), you create a climate of peace, and you do so without compromising your opinion or beliefs in any way. By accepting the person, you will find that all of the frustration, the anger and resentment you have been feeling simply ceases to exist. And you have not given up anything! Making it okay for them to say or do those things (and you may as well make it okay, it is going to happen anyway) eliminates the basis of controversy. There is simply nothing left to feel bad about. You need not agree, you need not accept what they do, you need only accept that person as a person who, like you, is a product of conditioning, doing what they have been conditioned to do, and believing what they have been conditioned to believe.

As humans, we seem to have a real and active need to be accepted by others. We sought acceptance as children and continue to do so as adults. We prefer to be with those who accept us and we seek them out. So, by accepting another, we make ourselves valuable to that other, and the other is then more apt to make himself more valuable to us. Thus, by accepting a 'recalcitrant other', you may well accomplish the change that you wanted in the first place. And, even if you do not accomplish the change, you will have achieved peace.

Acceptance must be communicated. If you accept another, it is necessary for the other to be aware that they are accepted if they and you are to benefit from it. And, if you accept, you cannot avoid communicating that acceptance. And, if you do not accept, you cannot avoid communicating rejection. Acceptance can be communicated in many ways: with words, by touching, listening, risking, trusting and by being non-defensive. You do none of those things with those you do not accept. Therefore, to do them is to communicate acceptance. And to not do them is to communicate rejection.

When you can say to another, "I can see that you feel strongly about that. I don't agree, and I wish you felt differently, but I understand that you don't," you are acknowledging the other as a responsible individual, doing so without compromising your own opinion. By acknowledging that they have a different opinion, you acknowledge that they have a right to hold that opinion and is therefore intelligent and worthy of your respect. By accepting, you enhance the other's self-image, perhaps setting the stage for acceptance of constructive criticism on their part.

It is not possible to fake acceptance. If you cannot actually and personally embrace the concept that the other person *is* doing, acting and believing as he must, then you will, without doing so consciously, make that fact known. The other person will sense it in many ways and will be resentful of your insincerity. If it is your desire to take the initiative, to bring harmony into a relationship, you can do so only if you can truly accept that person *as is*, making it okay for them to disagree with you, just as you disagree with them. If you can distinguish between the person and what the person does, you may be able to accept the person in spite of what they do and how you truly feel about it.

Acceptance is not for everyone. Of course, it may not be possible for you to accept a 'particular someone'. There are many people we do not accept, and that is okay too. We must be responsible to ourselves. We must defend ourselves and see that our own needs are met. However, if that particular someone is important and valuable, this concept of acceptance offers a way to draw that person closer. If acceptance is not possible, or if what that particular person is doing is truly intolerable, then it may be time to consider ending the relationship. Perhaps, by considering the relationship in that light, a new awareness of your own values will ensue. Both you and the other person have the power to heal and to bring harmony. Since you now know that you have the power, perhaps you should be the one to extend yourself.

Learning

When does learning begin? Why do we learn one thing rather than another from an experience? How can we relearn something in a different way? Can the change we seek to make be made by relearning? The answers to these questions are fundamental to the use of the technique, Subliminal Therapy.

Increasing evidence suggests that learning begins before birth, and the content of that learning has lifelong significance. Values, skills and behaviors are learned at all ages, and these lessons may be constructive or destructive, depending upon what we learned. Moreover, what we learn to be true today may be shown to be false tomorrow. A child, frightened in a dark place may learn to associate darkness with fear, and that learning, even though not appropriate in adult life, may have lifelong effect unless some form of relearning takes place.

It is accurate to say that we learned to walk, talk, read and do math. It is equally accurate to say that we learned to smoke, or to fear the dark or whatever it is that we wish to change now. Just as we learned something then, we can relearn it in a different way now. We have more information now than we had then. We know more about ourselves and about our world now than we did then. Subliminal Therapy will help to communicate that new learning to parts of the mind that are still functioning on the basis of past knowledge, parts that have not had opportunity to keep up with the rest of the mind.

This therapy emphasizes using unconscious abilities. However, whatever we do in the pursuit of change, we do by means of consciousness, motivated and instigated by conscious values and needs. Consciously desired change seems not to occur at all except as promoted by conscious will.

These most prevalent characteristics of consciousness (motivation and will) are not characteristics of the unconscious domain. Conversely, the most prevalent characteristics of the unconscious mind–memory, smooth muscle control, regulation of nonvoluntary physical functioning and a host of others – are not characteristics of the conscious domain. The capacity to reason, to form associations, to deduce and to recognize values, seem characteristic of both.

In my view, the unconscious mind is separate and independent of the conscious mind, not just a different function of a common mind. Different values, different needs, different strengths and different motivations seem to simultaneously exist in each of these domains. One indication of this difference is the commonly experienced dichotomy of thinking about things: "I know it's irrational to be afraid of the dark, but I am." "Of course I know I'm attractive, I just don't think I am." "I want to eat much less, but I eat more." However, I must emphasize that while such negative illustrations are true, it is also true that unconscious mental functioning is overwhelmingly positive and productive in the process of living. The following are examples of positive functioning of the unconscious mind, accomplished without the participation of consciousness in controlling the process:

- Walking and talking
- Writing
- Playing a musical instrument
- Regulation of digestion
- Regulation of glandular activity
- And more …

These, and all of the other thousands of things that require attention just to maintain life, are accomplished without conscious awareness. Therefore, they must be accomplished by the unconscious mind.

Skepticism

Mental growth consists of learning, of taking in new information and of becoming aware of new relationships between items of information we learn. In growing, we are presented with the need to learn new data, and we are also presented with the need to determine which items of the new data are valid. We must be skeptical. We must apply some test to the mass of ideas and information that is presented in order to judge what is right and what is wrong, what is true and what is false. We must test in order to separate reality from fantasy.

We must be skeptical to maintain a stable framework for coping with life. Without skepticism, that framework can be unduly shaken by new thoughts and ideas. Being skeptical, however, does not necessarily mean automatic rejection; it means critical evaluation. We must be open to the new to the extent of getting the information. Then, and only then, are we in a position to intelligently exercise critical judgment.

We often deny ourselves opportunity for growth by 'skeptically' avoiding exposure to information and understanding. In being skeptical, we sometimes shut out expressions of opposing views. We may also shut out all statements by an individual we expect will disagree with us. When this happens, whether done to avoid discomfort, to defend against attack, to avoid the possibility of being wrong or even without conscious awareness that we are doing so, a penalty is paid.

Another person may judge something as true that we judge as false. Someone else may be convinced of something that we consider absurd. Obviously, we and the other person are basing our opinions on different knowledge. We must, nevertheless, live by our own values, not another's values. We must make life's decisions on the basis of what we know, not on the basis of what another knows. Yet our knowledge is limited; the other just might be right. Perhaps it would be wise to consider what the other knows. Unless we are willing to risk exposure to a new and/or opposing viewpoint, we will never know.

Life consists of experiences. The greater the range and wealth of experience, the richer life becomes. We often have opportunities to have some experience, or to consider some idea or concept, that we avoid because of imagined risk. Yet, what of the risk of a limited life? Exploration need not be commitment.

Learned Dysfunction

We sometimes find ourselves doing or saying things that are inappropriate. Sometimes these things are serious and destructive; sometimes they are only minor annoyances or concerns. However, regardless of the degree of severity, these are learned behaviors. To illustrate, select some unwanted behavior of your own such as nail-biting. Look at its beginning and you will find that it began in some situation (first apparent), at some specific time (age ?), for some particular reason (nervousness). You were not born with it – it was learned.

As we mature, we learn all manner of skills, values and truths. We learn what is right and what is wrong. We learn what we can do, and we learn that there are limits to what we can do. Sometimes the limits we learn are false limits, limits that are based on false information or on misunderstanding, and those limits become just as real as other limits ("I can't cook, I can't even boil an egg"). Such false limits may relate to physical strength or endurance; they may also relate to mental capacities such as memory or intelligence.

As we mature, most of what we learn is positive. We learn to walk and talk. We learn to love and to cope with life in productive ways. Yet, sometimes we learn false, negative or dysfunctional behaviors. We may have learned to get our way by a display of temper, and we may have internalized that as a way of coping generally, even as adults. We may have learned to fear something irrationally, or to express our emotions in physical ways that become the physical dysfunctions we now identify as illness.

To understand this last point, consider the close correlation between what we experience emotionally and what we experience physically. As I previously mentioned, when we experience anger or fear, the pattern of blood flow within our body changes, digestion ceases, glandular function is altered, blood chemistry changes and a long list of other changes take place. All negative emotions produce negative (dysfunctional) physical responses. Positive emotions produce positive (healthy) physical responses.

Moreover, prolonged experience of negative emotion can produce physical illness, even if the emotion is only experienced unconsciously.

Examples of how unconscious experiences, beliefs, emotions and thoughts can impact us physically are numerous. For instance, if we repress an emotion, rather than expressing it in a functional way, we will unconsciously express it in a dysfunctional way. Suppressed grief may emerge as the 'crying' of hay fever, suppressed fear may emerge as colitis, suppressed vocalizing as stuttering, anger as arthritis, tension as ulcers and guilt as headaches.

Smooth muscle systems, under the control of the unconscious domain of the mind, provide the mechanics of these physical reactions. These muscle systems control the pattern of blood flow, glandular activity, digestion and the thousands of other activities that go on without ceasing and without conscious awareness, to maintain life. These systems are influenced by the unconscious experiences, beliefs and emotions that are a product of life's conditioning. Moreover, such influence may be functional or dysfunctional.

Whether we express an emotion in a functional way, or repress it and then express it in a dysfunctional way, depends upon how we learned to express it in the first place. When we learned to express it, it was rational that we would have learned to do so as we did, even though it may appear irrational in the light of present knowledge. For example, if we learned to fear the dark, it was in circumstances in which it was logical to be afraid and it was logical that we would have formed an association between fear and dark. Similarly, if we experienced pain and gained attention because of it, we might later continue to experience pain for that learned (now unconscious) reason. And we might do so despite conscious desire to change. In this way, the problem of today was the solution to a problem of yesterday.

The process of learning things may be conscious, as might occur in a schoolroom, or it may be without conscious awareness. In either event, it is important to know that learning was involved, because anything that has been learned in one way can be relearned in a different way, with different consequences.

A few examples of dysfunctions that may have been learned are listed below. In each of these examples, relearning of appropriate response is likely to be possible.

- Hard to get up
- Neck and shoulder pain
- Irritability
- Snoring
- Limits to learning
- Morning sickness
- Phobias
- Sexual dysfunction
- Depression
- Low back pain
- Headaches
- Thumb sucking
- Torticollis
- Asthma
- Stuttering
- Hay fever
- Tics
- Colitis
- Hyper-gagging
- Ulcers

Suggestibility

When we are exposed to a new idea or concept, we will normally consider it in the light of what we already know about this and related subjects. We will believe or disbelieve, accept or reject, on that basis. In other words, we exercise critical judgment about it. Sometimes, however, our critical judgment is bypassed, and then the new idea or concept can become internalized without being critically judged. At these times we are said to be 'suggestible'.

We are spontaneously suggestible in several situations, sometimes when not even consciously aware that learning is taking place. In illustration, the person who stutters was probably conditioned to stutter without being aware, consciously, that the conditioning was taking place. In other words, the person perceived the conditioning influence unconsciously and it was integrated by the unconscious, without conscious awareness that it was happening.

We are highly suggestible when we are very young, before we have accumulated sufficient knowledge as the basis for critical judgment. A small child will believe anything presented, unless there is prior knowledge to the contrary. For this reason, it is important to limit the child's exposure, to protect the child from undesirable influence. As the child matures, the accumulation of knowledge permits critical judgment, thereby diminishing suggestibility and the need for protection.

People are suggestible when experiencing hypnosis. Yet, while that seems to be true, it is qualified. People are *more* suggestible, but only about some things, at some times, in some situations. In other words, it is not an all-or-nothing condition. Yet people are more suggestible when experiencing hypnosis. This is a characteristic of the state that lends it authority to influence us, whether for good or for ill.

Another condition of life in which people are suggestible is when experiencing intense emotion. It seems not to matter what emotion is involved; it may be fear, anger, joy, grief or any other emotion. Moreover, the greater the intensity of the emotional experience, the greater the degree of suggestibility experienced. A varied assortment of dysfunctions may be incurred in this condition; sexual problems, stuttering, tics and phobias are common examples.

Suggestibility also accompanies confusion. Not only do people make mistakes when confused, they may also unconsciously accept suggestions, and thereby integrate them, when confused. Whether those suggestions are intentionally presented (as sometimes employed in sales techniques), or whether they are coincidental, they may have long-term effect.

Some suggestions are internalized at a level that permits easy replacement by preferred suggestions; other suggestions seem to be internalized at more profound levels and resist replacement. The extreme of such internalization is called 'imprinting', an experience usually limited to childhood or to intense trauma. Moreover, it seems that the degree to which suggestions are internalized is determined by the degree of suggestibility in effect at the time of exposure to the suggestion.

In learning, one suggestion may replace another as the person identifies and understands the first in the light of current knowledge. They may then permit new decisions about the original situation. This capacity makes change possible.

Sex

Sex! The very word commands attention. It is the most intimate of human experiences, the favorite topic of humor low and high, the subject most commonly occupying our thoughts and the subject least likely to be discussed freely in our culture, though most in need of discussion. It is almost as though taboos preclude discussion of those matters which warrant such discussion most. Sex is too important not to talk about! Ignorance and misinformation about sex produce much unnecessary guilt, fear and unhappiness.

We are sexual creatures. We are born so and we remain so until death. Children commonly learn at a very early age that genital touch is pleasurable. That pleasure response continues through life. This is our nature; it is the way we were created. To be ignorant of this essential aspect of our nature, or to deny it, is to invite unhappiness. To be informed about it is to open doors to one of life's most fulfilling experiences. Here I will present several aspects of our sexuality in an abruptly open fashion, thereby opening wide the doors of discussion.

The Beauty of Sex

The sexual act is the most intimate experience available to us; no other aspect of our lives is so charged with emotional energy. To be sure, we have a physical aspect of sex; it feels good! It is enjoyable and apparently was intended to be enjoyed. However, we also have the potential of even further value when sex is used to *give* pleasure, as well as to *receive* it and when it is used to communicate loving regard. It is in these instances that the act of sexual contact takes on an element of beauty unknown to many in our culture.

Sexual freedom increases with each generation (to the frequent dismay of the preceding generation), and I see this increase as beneficial. The general promiscuity past generations feared has not materialized, and the accompanying exposure of the realities of our sexuality relieves many of us from unnecessary guilt, fear and consequent unhappiness. Our sexuality is a God-given fact of life and was apparently meant to be enjoyed. We can enjoy it more, and enjoy it more responsibly, if we are informed about it!

Consequences of Ignorance

Guilt and apprehension are frequent consequences of childhood and adolescent exposures of a sexual nature. Sexual curiosity is often satisfied by mutual exploration. Playing doctor is frequently our first form of sex education. This education, shrouded in secrecy, may leave the participants feeling guilty or with their self-image compromised. Such experiences, when involving mutual masturbation between members of the same sex, may result in serious misgivings about personal sexuality or even sexual identity. Unless someone provides awareness that such activity is typical and neither unnatural nor deviant, such consequences may be lifelong in duration.

We also need knowledge about how easily we can be stimulated sexually. Both young and old are sometimes confused and dismayed by unexpected erotic feelings that are both natural and understandable. While we can be sexually stimulated by a member of the opposite sex, as our culture says is 'normal', we can also be stimulated by a member of the same sex, or by an animal, a machine or by our own imagination. This is the reality of our sexuality. When we understand this, we can avoid much unhappiness. Until we understand this, it seems unhappiness is inevitable.

Another illustration of unnecessary unhappiness resulting from our reluctance to discuss sexual issues, is the unfortunate schism between father and daughter that may occur as the daughter enters adolescence. Such result is the consequence of misunderstanding born of ignorance about sexual response. She is becoming aware of her sexuality in many ways; her body is developing and members of the opposite sex are noticing her in unaccustomed ways. And she may test that sexuality by developing mannerisms that accent it. From the father's perspective, the cuddly little darling of so many romps and loving contacts is suddenly recognized as a sexual being, a recognition that prompts a biological response in him which must be controlled. Since these feelings cannot be denied, and since they all too often cannot be admitted, he may cope by keeping his daughter at a distance, avoiding contact, thereby keeping his feelings in check. His daughter, being unaware of his dilemma, may perceive his actions as rejection, inexplicable and frequently resented rejection, and may react accordingly. On the other hand, with understanding of the normalcy of his reaction, the father can establish safeguards. Then they can continue a close, loving relationship.

Masturbation

The best data available indicate that well over 90 percent of all males, and in excess of 60 percent of all females, masturbate – not just in adolescence, but throughout life. Yet, since social conventions forbid discussion of this natural activity, we may unnecessarily feel guilt or apprehension for having masturbated. Some religious persuasions teach that masturbation is a sin, thereby guaranteeing guilt for most of their followers. When children are discovered in some exploration of a sexual nature, parents often communicate censure and induce guilt. The same covert message comes from other sources as well. All such messages fly in the face of reality – the reality of the normal humanness of the act. Assuming no guilt or fear results, masturbation is natural and without harm to self or others.

Many persons not involved in an intimate relationship are caught between the biological demand for sexual expression and cultural restrictions. For such persons, recognition of the normalcy of masturbation can make it possible to satisfy the biological need without consequent guilt.

Sexual Molestation

Tragically, sexual molestation of children by adults is all too common. Not that actual intercourse or physical injury necessarily occurs, although it often does, but rather seductive contact and erotic stimulation takes place in a secretive way. Such an experience can emotionally scar a child in lasting ways which interfere with a fulfilling expression of sexuality, and which can be far more damaging than physical scars.

If the emotional scar takes the form of guilt, it is likely that the guilt is not the result of actions engaged in, but rather from the enjoyment of the feelings experienced. Because of the secretive ways it happens, the child is aware that there is something wrong with what is happening, and may conclude that the undeniable pleasure from the genital contact is also wrong. Intelligent discussion of the event, in which the normalcy of the experience of pleasure is exposed, is perhaps the only way of resolving the resultant guilt. For the benefit of the child, the sooner such discussion can occur, the better.

If the emotional scar takes the form of fear of sexual expression, the individual is denied this rich and fulfilling aspect of life. And, finally, if the emotional scar takes the form of bitterness at having been mistreated, the individual may be prevented from forming close relationships with the opposite sex, or may have no interest in experiencing sex at all. As I have discussed elsewhere in this book, bitterness is insidious, and its effects tend to spread into other areas.

References and Further Reading

Ahmad, A., Larsson, B. & Sundelin-Wahlsten, V. (2007). EMDR treatment for children with PTSD: results of a randomized controlled trial. *Nordic Journal of Psychiatry*, 61 (5), 349–354.

Allington, H.V. (1952). Review of the psychotherapy of warts. *Archives of Dermatology and Syphilogy*, 66 (3), 316–326.

American Medical Association, Council on Scientific Affairs (1985). Scientific status of refreshing recollection by the use of hypnosis. *Journal of the American Medical Association*, 253 (13), 1918–1923.

Anbar, R.D. (2003). Automatic word processing: a new forum for hypnotic expression. *American Journal of Clinical Hypnosis*, 44 (1), 27–36.

Anbar, R.D. (2008). Subconscious guided therapy with hypnosis. *American Journal of Clinical Hypnosis*, 50 (3), 323–334.

Assagioli, R. (1965). *Psychosynthesis*. New York: Penguin Books.

Augustynek, A. (1977). Recalling in a state of awareness and under hypnosis. *Przeglad Psychologiciczny*, 20, 82–84.

Augustynek, A., with Haynes, B. & Patrick, B.S. (1983). Hypnosis, memory and incidental memory. *Journal of the American Society of Clinical Hypnosis*, 25 (4), 253–262.

Augustynek, A., with Patrick, B.S. (1987). Hypnosis and memory: the effects of emotional arousal. *Journal of the American Society of Clinical Hypnosis*, 29, 177–184.

Bandler, R. & Grinder, J. (1975). *Patterns of the Hypnotic Techniques of Milton. H. Erickson, M.D.* Cupertino, CA: Meta Publishing.

Bandler, R. & Grinder, J. (1979). *Frogs into Princes: Neuro Linguistic Programming*. Moab, UT: Real People Press.

Bandler, R. & Grinder, J. (1983). *Reframing: Neuro-Linguistic Programming and the Transformation of Meaning*. Moab, UT: Real People Press.

Barsky, A., Saintfort, R., Rogers, M. & Borus, J. (2002). Nonspecific medication side effects and the nocebo phenomenon. *Journal of the American Medical Association*, 287 (5), 622–627.

Bellamy R. (1997). Compensation neurosis: financial reward for illness as nocebo. *Clinical Orthopedics and Related Research*, 336, 94–106.

Beneditti, F. (2003). Conscious expectation and unconscious conditioning in analgesic, motor and harmonal placebo/nocebo responses. *Journal of Neuroscience*, 23 (10), 4315–4323.

Bennett, H.L. (1988). Perception and memory for events during adequate general anesthesia for surgical operations. In H.M. Pettinati (ed.), *Hypnosis and Memory* (pp. 193–231). New York: Guilford.

Bloomgarden, A. & Calogero, R.M. (2008). A randomized experimental test of the efficacy of EMDR treatment on negative body image in eating disorder inpatients. *Eating Disorders*, 16 (5), 418–427.

Bowers, K.S. (1976). *Hypnosis for the Seriously Curious*. New York: Norton.

Bresler, D.E. (1990). Meeting an inner advisor. In: D.C. Hammond (ed.), *Handbook of Hypnotic Suggestions and Metaphors* (pp. 318–320). New York: W.W. Norton.

Cannon, W.B. (1953). *Bodily Changes in Pain, Hunger, Fear, and Rage: An Account of Recent Researches into the Function of Emotional Excitement.* Boston, MA: Branford.

Chamberlain, D.B. (1986). Reliability of birth memory: observations from mother and child pairs in hypnosis. *Journal of the American Academy of Medical Hypnoanalysts*, 1 (2), 89–98.

Chamberlain, D.B. (1988). *Babies Remember birth*. Los Angeles, CA: Tarcher.

Cheek, D.B. (1975). Maladjustment patterns apparently related to imprinting at birth. *Journal of the American Society of Clinical Hypnosis*, 18 (2), 75–82.

Cheek, D.B. (1974). Sequential head and shoulder movements appearing with age regression in hypnosis to birth. *Journal of the American Society of Clinical Hypnosis*, 16 (4), 261–266.

Cheek, D.B. (1994). *Hypnosis: The Application of Ideomotor Techniques.* Boston, MA: Allyn & Bacon.

Cheek, D.B. & LeCron, L.M. (1968). *Clinical Hypnotherapy*. New York: Grune & Stratton.

Clavel-Chapelon, F., Paoletti, C. & Benhamou, S. (1997). Smoking cessation rates 4 years after treatment by nicotine gum and acupuncture. *Preventive Medicine*, 26 (1), 25–28.

Clawson, T.A. & Swade, R.H. (1975). The hypnotic control of blood flow and pain: the cure of warts and the potential for the use of hypnosis in the treatment of cancer. *Journal of the American Society of Clinical Hypnosis*, 17 (3), 160–169.

Clemens, S.L. (1884). *Huckleberry Finn*. New York: C.L. Webster.

Cohen, S.B. (1978). Warts. *Journal of the American Society of Clinical Hypnosis*, 20 (3), 165–174.

Cooper, L.M. (1966). Spontaneous and suggested post-hypnotic source amnesia. *International Journal of Clinical and Experimental Hypnosis*, 14 (2), 180–193.

Coventry, P.A. & Gellatly, J.L. (2007). Improving outcomes for COPD patients with mild-to-moderate anxiety and depression: a systematic review of cognitive behavioral therapy. *British Journal of Health Psychology*, 13 (3), 381–400.

Crawford, H.L. & Allen, S.N. (1983). Enhanced visual memories during hypnosis as mediated by hypnotic responsiveness and cognitive strategies. *Journal of Experimental Psychology: General*, 112 (4), 662–685.

DePiano, F.A. & Salzberg, H.C. (1981). Hypnosis as an aid to recall of meaningful information presented under three types of arousal. *International Journal of Clinical and Experimental Hypnosis*, 29, 383–400.

Dhanens, T.P. & Lundy, R.M. (1975). Hypnosis and waking suggestions and recall. *International Journal of Clinical and Experimental Hypnosis*, 23, 68–79.

Dinges, D.F., Whitehouse, W.G., Orne, E.C., Powell, J.W., Orne, M.T. & Erdelyi, M.H. (1992). Hypnotic memory enhancement (hypermnesia and reminiscence) using multitrial forced recall. *Journal of Experimental Psychology*, 18 (5), 1139–1147.

Dywan, L. & Bowers, K.S. (1983). The use of hypnosis to enhance recall. *Science*, 222, 184–185.

Echterling, L.G. & Emmerling, D.A. (1987). Impact of stage hypnosis. *Journal of the American Society of Clinical Hypnosis*, 29 (3), 149–154.

Edmond, T., Rubin, A. & Wambach, K. (1999). The effectiveness of EMDR with adult female survivors of childhood sexual abuse. *Social Work Research*, 23 (2), 103–116.

Elman, D. (1964). *Explorations in Hypnosis*. Los Angeles, CA: Nash.

Erdelyi, M.H. (1988). Hypermnesia: the effect of hypnosis, fantasy, and concentration. In M. Pettinati (ed.), *Hypnosis and Memory* (pp. 64–90). New York: Guilford.

Esdale, J. (1850). *Hypnosis in Medicine and Surgery*. New York: Julian.

Erickson, M.H. (1937). Development of apparent unconsciousness during hypnotic reliving of a traumatic event. *Archives of Neurology & Psychiatry*, 38, 1282–1288.

Erickson, M.H. (1960). Breast development possibly influenced by hypnosis: two instances of and the therapeutic results. *Journal of the American Society of Clinical Hypnosis*, 2 (3), 157–159.

Erickson, M.H. (1989a). Basic psychological problems in hypnotic research. In E.L. Rossi (ed.), *The Collected Papers of Milton H. Erickson on Hypnosis, Vol. II.* (pp. 340–350). New York: Irvington.

Erickson, M.H. (1989b). Hypnotherapeutic approaches to rehabilitation. In E.L. Rossi (ed.), *The Collected Papers of Milton H. Erickson, Vol. IV* (pp. 306–371). New York: Irvington.

Erickson, M.H. & Rossi, E.L. (1976). *Hypnotic Realities*. New York: Irvington.

Erickson, M.H. & Rossi, E.L. (1979). *Hypnotherapy: An Exploratory Casebook*. New York: Irvington.

Ewin, D. (1992). Hypnotherapy for warts. *Journal of the American Society of Clinical Hypnosis*, 35 (1), 1–10.

Ewin, D. (2006). *Ideomotor Signals for Rapid Hypnoanalysis*. Springfield, IL: Charles C. Thomas.

Evans, F.J. (1988). Post-hypnotic amnesia: dissociation of content and context. In H.M. Pettinati (ed.), *Hypnosis and Memory* (pp. 157–190). New York: Guilford.

Evans, F.J. & Thorn, W.A.F. (1966). Two types of post-hypnotic amnesia: recall amnesia and source amnesia. *International Journal of Clinical and Experimental Hypnosis*, 14, 162–179.

Frankel, F.H. (1988). The clinical use of hypnosis in aiding recall. In H.M. Pettinati (ed.), *Hypnosis and memory* (pp. 247–264). New York: Guilford.

Freud, S. (1938). *General Psychological Theory: Papers on Metapsychology*. Sutton Valence, Kent: Touchstone Books 2008.

Gheorg, V. (1967). Some peculiarities of post-hypnotic source amnesia of information. In L. Chertok (ed.), *Psychophysiological Mechanisms in Hypnosis* (pp. 112–122). New York: Springer.

Grainger, R., Levin, C., Allen-Byrd, L., Doctor, R. & Lee, H. (1997). An empirical evaluation of eye movement desensitization and reprocessing (EMDR) with survivors of a natural disaster. *Journal of Traumatic Stress*, 10 (4), 665–671.

Gravitz, M.A. (1981). The production of warts by suggestion as a cultural phenomenon. *Journal of the American Society of Clinical Hypnosis*, 23 (4), 281–283.

Green, E. & Green, A. (1977). *Beyond Biofeedback*. New York: Dell.

Grinder, J. & Bandler, R. (1981). *Trance-Formations*. Moab, UT: Real People Press.

Hahn, R.A. (1997). The nocebo phenomenon: the concept, evidence and implications for public health. *Preventive Medicine*, 26 (5), 607–611.

Haley, J. (1967). *Advanced Techniques of Hypnosis and Therapy*. New York: Grune & Stratton.

Haley, J. (1973). *Uncommon Therapy*. New York: Norton.

Hendriks G.J., Oude Voshaar R.C., Keijsers G.P., Hoogduin C.A. & van Balkom, A.J. (2008). Cognitive-behavioural therapy for late-life anxiety disorders: a systematic review and meta-analysis. *Acta Psychiatrica Scandinavica*, 117 (6), 403–411.

Hilgard, E.R. (1978a). A neodissociation interpretation of pain reduction in hypnosis. *Psychological Review*, 80, 396–394.

Hilgard, E.R. (1978b). *Divided Consciousness*. New York: Wiley.

Hull, C.L. (1933). *Hypnosis and Suggestibility*. New York: Appleton.

Hunter, R. (2005). *Hypnosis for Inner Conflict Resolution: Introducing Parts Therapy*. Carmarthen, Wales: Crown House Publishing.

Hynninen, M.J., Bjerke, N., Pallesen, S., Bakke, P.S. & Nordhus, I.H. (2010). A randomized controlled trial of cognitive behavioral therapy for anxiety and depression in COPD. *Respiratory Medicine*, 104 (7), 986–994.

Ironson, G., Freund, B. & Strauss, J.L. (2002). Comparison of two treatments for traumatic stress: a community-based study of EMDR and prolonged exposure. *Journal of Clinical Psychology*, 58 (1), 113–128.

Jaberghaderi, N., Greenwald, R., Rubin, A., Dolatabadim S. & Zand, S.O. (2004). A comparison of CBT and EMDR for sexually abused Iranian girls. *Clinical Psychology and Psychotherapy*, 11, 358–368.

Jackson, E.N. (1947). *Understanding Grief*. New York: Wiley.

James, W. (1890). *Principles of Psychology*. New York: Holt.

Janet, P. (1907). *Major Symptoms of Hysteria*. New York: MacMillan.

Johnson, R.F.Q. & Barber, T.X. (1978). Hypnosis, suggestion and warts: an experimental investigation implicating the importance of 'believed-in efficacy'. *Journal of the American Society of Clinical Hypnosis*, 20 (3), 165–174.

Jung, C. G. (1916) *The Psychology of the Unconscious*. New York: Dover Publications.

Jung, C.G. (1933). *Modern Man in Search of a Soul*. New York: Harcourt Brace.

Keller, M.B., McCullough, J.P., Klien, D.N., Dunnder, D.L. & Gelenberg, A.J. (2000). A comparison of nefazodone, the cognitive-behavioral analysis system of psychotherapy, and their combination for the treatment of chronic depression. *New England Journal of Medicine*, 342, 1462–1470.

Klienhauz, M. & Beran, B. (1984). Misuse of hypnosis: a factor in psychopathology. *Journal of the American Society of Clinical Hypnosis*, 26 (4), 283–290.

Klienhauz, M. & Eli, H. (1987). Potential deleterious effect of hypnosis in the clinical setting. *Journal of the American Society of Clinical Hypnosis*, 29 (3), 155–159.

Kline, M.V. (1955). *Hypnodynamic Psychology*. New York: Julian Press.

Kroger, W.S. (1963). *Clinical and Experimental Hypnosis*. Philadelphia, PA: Lippincott.

Kroger, W.S. (1976). *Hypnosis and Behavior Modification: Imagery Conditioning*. New York: Lippincott.

Kroger, W.S. & Douce, R.G. (1979). Hypnosis in criminal investigation. *International Journal of Clinical and Experimental Hypnosis*, 27 (4), 358–374.

Kroger, W.S. & Douce, R.G. (1980). Forensic use of hypnosis. *Journal of the American Society of Clinical Hypnosis*, 23 (2), 73–118.

LaMaze, F. (1965). *Painless Childbirth*. New York: Pocket Books.

LeCron, L.M. (1965). *Experimental Hypnosis*. New York: Citadel.

LeCron, L.M. (1972). A study of age regression under hypnosis. In L.M. LeCron (ed.), *Experimental Hypnosis* (pp. 155–177). New York: Citadel.

Linder, R.M. (1952). Hypnoanalysis. In R. Rhodes (ed.), *Therapy Through Hypnosis* (pp. 213–231). New York: Citidel.

MacHovee, F. (1988). Hypnosis complications: six cases, risk factors and prevention. *Journal of the American Society of Clinical Hypnosis*, 31 (1), 40–49.

MacHovee, F. & Oster, M. (1999). In the best of families. *Journal of the American Society of Clinical Hypnosis*, 42 (1), 3–9.

MacHovee, M.A. (1997). Complications following hypnosis in a psychotic patient with sexual dysfunction treated by a lay hypnotist. *Journal of the American Society of Clinical Hypnosis*, 29 (3), 166–170.

Magnuson, R.L. (1984). Pain control. In G. Pratt, D. Wood & B. Alman (eds.), *A Clinical Hypnosis Primer* (pp. 173–186). La Jolla, CA: Psychology and Counseling Associates Press.

Mears, A. (1961). An evaluation of the dangers of medical hypnosis. *Journal of the American Society of Clinical Hypnosis*, 4 (2), 90–97.

Melzac, R. & Wall, P. (1965). *The Challenge of Pain*. New York: Penguin.

Morris, B.A.P. (1985). Hypnotic treatment of warts using the Simonton visualization technique: a case report. *Journal of the American Society of Clinical Hypnosis*, 27 (4), 237–240.

Norton, P.J. & Price, E.C. (2007). A meta-analytic review of adult cognitive-behavioral treatment outcome across the anxiety disorders. *Journal of Nervous and Mental Disease*, 195 (6), 521–531.

NyQuist, O. (1986). Breast enlargement by hypnosis: a self-concept variable. Unpublished doctoral dissertation, Professional School of Psychological Studies, San Diego, CA.

Orne, M.T., Soskis, D.A., Dinges, D.G. & Orne, E.C. (1984). Hypnotically induced testimony and the criminal justice system. In G.L. Wells & E.F. Loftus (eds.), *Advances in the Psychology of Eyewitness Testimony* (pp. 171–213). New York: Cambridge University Press.

Penfield, W. (1975). *The Mystery of the Mind.* Princeton, NJ: Princeton University Press.

Perry, C.W., Laurence, J.R., D'eon, J. & Jallant, B. (1988). Hypnotic age regression techniques in the elicitation of memories: applied uses and abuses. In H.M. Pettinati (ed.), *Hypnosis and Memory* (pp. 128–148). New York: Guilford.

Pettinati, H.M. (1988). Hypnosis and memory: Integrative summary and future directions. In H.M. Pettinati (ed.), *Hypnosis and Memory* (pp. 277–289). New York: Guilford.

Pigott, H.E., Levanthal, A.M., Alter, G.S. & Boren, J.J. (2010). Efficacy and effectiveness of antidepressants: current status of research. *Psychotherapy and Psychosomatics*, 79, 267–279.

Podvill, E.M. & Goodman, S.J. (1949). The effect of relaxation on recall. *American Journal of Psychology*, 62, 33–47.

Pratt, G.J., Wood, D.P. & Alman, B.M. (1984). *A Clinical Hypnosis Primer.* La Jolla, CA: PCA Press.

Puffer, M.K., Greenwald, R. & Elrod, D.E. (1998). A single session EMDR study with twenty traumatized children and adolescents. *The International Electronic Journal of Innovations in the Study of the Traumatization Process and Methods for Reducing or Eliminating Related Human Suffering*, 3:2, Article 6.

Putman, W.H. (1979). Hypnosis and distortions in eyewitness memory. *International Journal of Clinical and Experimental Hypnosis*, 27 (4), 437–448.

Quackenbos, J. (1908). *Hypnotic Therapeutics in Theory and Practice.* New York: Harper.

Raikov, V.L. (1980). Age regression to infancy by adult subjects in deep hypnosis. *Journal of the American Society of Clinical Hypnosis*, 22 (3), 156–163.

Raikov, V.L. (1982). Hypnotic age regression to the neonatal period: comparison with role playing. *Journal of the American Society of Clinical Hypnosis*, 30 (2), 108–116.

Rector, N.A., Cassin, S.E. and Rector, M.A (2009). Psychological treatment of obsessive-compulsive disorder in patients with major depression: a pilot randomized controlled study. *Canadian Journal of Psychiatry*, 54 (12), 846–851.

Reiser, M. (1976). Hypnosis as a tool in criminal investigation. In *"The Police Chief" Handbook of Investigating Hypnosis*. (1980). Los Angeles, CA: Law Enforcement Hypnosis Institute.

Reiser, M. (1980). *Handbook of Investigative Hypnosis*. Los Angeles, CA: LEHI Publishing Co.

Reiser, M. (1982). *Police Psychology Collected Papers*. Los Angeles, CA: LEHI Publishing Co.

Reiser, M. & Nielson, M. (1980). Investigative hypnosis: a developing specialty. *Journal of the American Society of Clinical Hypnosis*, 23 (2), 75–85.

Relinger, H. (1984). Hypnotic hypermnesia: a critical review. *Journal of the American Society of Clinical Hypnosis*, 26 (3), 212–225.

Rezvan, S., Baghban, I., Bahrami, F. & Abedi, M. (2008). A comparison of cognitive-behavioral therapy with interpersonal and cognitive behavior therapy in the treatment of generalized anxiety disorder. *Counseling Psychology Quarterly*, 21 (4), 309–321.

Rhodes, R.N. (1952). *Therapy through Hypnosis*. New York: Citadel.

Rogers, C.R. (1951). *Client Centered Therapy*. New York: Houghton Mifflin.

Rosenthal, B.G. (1944). Hypnotic recall of material learned under anxiety and non-anxiety producing conditions. *Journal of Experimental Psychology*, 34, 369–389.

Roy-Byrne, P.P., Craske, M.G., Stein, M.B., Sullivan, G., Bystritsky, S., Kanton, W., Golinelli, D. & Sherbourne, C. (2004). A randomized effectiveness trial of cognitive-behavioral therapy and medication for primary care panic disorder. *Archives of General Psychiatry* 62 (3), 290–298.

Schafer, D.W. & Rubio, R. (1978). Hypnosis to aid the recall of witnesses. *International Journal of Clinical and Experimental Hypnosis*, 26 (2), 81–91.

Sears, A.B. (1978). A comparison of hypnotic and waking recall. *International Journal of Clinical and Experimental Hypnosis*, 2 (4), 296–304.

Scheck, M.M., Schaeffer, J.A. & Gillette, C. (1998). Brief psychological intervention with traumatized young women: the efficacy of eye movement desensitization and reprocessing. *Journal of Traumatic Stress*, 11 (1), 25–44.

Sheehan, D.V. (1978). Influence of psychosocial factors in wart remission. *Journal of the American Society of Clinical Hypnosis*, 20 (3), 160–164.

Shields, I.W. & Knox, J. (1986). Level of processing as a determinant in hypnotic hypermnesia. *Journal of Abnormal Psychology*, 95 (4), 358–364.

Sinclair-Gieben, A.H.C. & Chalmers, D. (1959). Evaluation of treatment of warts by hypnosis. *The Lancet*, 2, 480–482.

Spanos, N.P., Gwynn, M.L, Comer, S.L., Baltruweit, W.J. & de Groh, M. (1989). Are hypnotically induced psuedomemories resistant to cross-examination? *Law and Behavior*, 13 (3), 271–289.

Spiegel, H. (1997). Nocebo: the power of suggestibility. *Preventive Medicine*, 26 (5), 616–621.

Spinhoven, P. & Wijk J. (1992). Hypnotic age regression in an experimental and clinical context. *Journal of the American Society of Clinical Hypnosis*, 35 (1), 40–46.

Stager, G.L. & Lundy, R.M. (1985). Hypnosis and the learning and recall of visually presented material. *International Journal of Clinical and Experimental Hypnosis*, 33, 27–39.

Staib, A.R. & Logan, D.R. (1997). Hypnotic stimulation of breast growth. *Journal of the American Society of Clinical Hypnosis*, 19 (4), 201–208.

Stalnaker, J.M. & Riddle, E.E. (1932). The effect of hypnosis on long-delayed recall. *Journal of General Psychology*, 6, 429–440.

Stankler, L. (1967). A critical assessment of the cure of warts by suggestion. *Practitioner*, 198, 690–694.

Stein, C. (1963). The clenched fist technique as a hypnotic procedure in clinical psychotherapy. *Journal of the American Society of Clinical Hypnosis*, 5 (2), 113–119.

Stone, H. & Winkelman S. (1989). *Embracing Ourselves: The Voice Dialogue Manual*. San Rafael, CA: New World Library.

Stratton, L.G. (1977). The use of hypnosis in law enforcement: a pilot program. *Journal of Police Science and Administration*, 5 (4), 399–406.

Strickler, C.B. (1929). A quantitative study of post-hypnotic amnesia. *Journal of Abnormal Social Psychology*, 24, 108–119.

Surman, O.S., Gottlieb, S.K. & Hackett, T.P. (1972). Hypnotic treatment of a child with warts. *Archives of General Psychiatry*, 28, 439–441.

Tasini, M.F. & Hackett, T.F. (1977). Hypnosis in the treatment of warts in immunodeficient children. *Journal of the American Society of Clinical Hypnosis*, 19 (3), 152–154.

Tenzel, J.F. & Taylor, R.H. (1969). An evaluation of hypnosis and suggestion as treatment for warts. *Psychosomatics*, 10, 252–257.

Thomas, L. (1979). *The Medusa and the Snail*. New York: Penguin.

True, R.M. (1949). Experimental control in hypnotic age regression states. *Science*, 2 (110), 583–584.

Turner, E.H., Matthews, S.M., Linardatos, E., Tell, R.A. & Rosenthal, R. (2008). Selective publication of antidepressant trials and its influence on apparent efficacy. *New England Journal of Medicine*, 358, 252–260.

Ulman, M. (1959). On the psyche and warts: suggestion and warts, a review and comments. *Psychosomatic Medicine*, 21, 473–488.

Wain, H.J. (1980). *Clinical Hypnosis in Medicine*. Chicago, IL: Year Book Medical Publishers.

Watkins, H.H. (1993). Ego state therapy: an overview. *American Journal of Clinical Hypnosis*, 35, 232–240.

Watkins, J.G. (1949). *Hypnotherapy of War Neuroses*. New York: Ronald Press.

Watkins, J.G. (1978). *The Therapeutic Self*. New York: Human Sciences.

Watkins, J.G. (1989). Hypnotic hypermnesia and forensic hypnosis: a cross examination. *Journal of the American Society of Clinical Hypnosis*, 32 (2), 71–83.

Watkins, J.G. & Watkins, H.H. (1979). Ego states and hidden observers. *Journal of Altered States of Consciousness*, 5 (3), 18.

Webster, W.C. (1987). *Clinical Hypnosis*. Cincinnati, OH: Behavioral Sciences Center.

Weitzenhoffer, A.M. (1957). *General Techniques of Hypnotism*. New York: Grune & Stratton.

Whitaker, R. (2010). *Anatomy of an Epidemic: Magic Bullets, Psychiatric Drugs, and the Astonishing Rise of Mental Illness in America*. New York: Crown Publishing Group/Random House.

White, R.W., Fox, G.F. & Harris, W.W. (1940). Hypnotic hypermnesia for recently learned material. *Journal of Abnormal Social Psychology*, 35, 88–103.

Willard, R.D. (1977). Breast enlargement through visual imagery and hypnosis. *Journal of the American Society of Clinical Hypnosis*, 19 (4), 195–200.

Williams, R.M. (2004). *The Missing Peace In Your Life!* Crestone, CO: Myrddin Publications.

Williams, R.M. (2008). *PSYCH-K: The Missing Peace In Your Life!* Crestone, CO: Myrddin Publications.

Wolberg, L.R. (1948). *Medical Hypnosis*. New York: Grune & Stratton.

Wolberg, L.R. (1945). *Hypnoanalysis*. New York: Grune & Stratton.

Wolf, S. (1950). Effects of suggestion and conditioning on the action of chemical agents in human subjects: the pharmacology of placebos. *Journal of Clinical Investigation*, 29 (1), 100–109.

Yager, E.K. (1978). *Subliminal Therapy: Utilizing Unconscious Abilities in Therapy*. Self-published.

Yager, E.K. (1985). *Subliminal Therapy: Utilizing the Unconscious Mind*. Self-published.

Yager, E.K. (1987). Subliminal therapy: utilizing the unconscious mind. *Journal of the American Academy of Medical Hypnoanalysts*, 11 (4), 156–160.

Yager, E.K. (2002). Hypnosis in criminal investigation. *The Law Enforcement Quarterly*, 31 (2), published by the Office of the District Attorney, County of San Diego.

Yager, E.K. (2008). *Foundations of Clinical Hypnosis: From Theory to Practice*. Carmarthen, Wales: Crown House Publishing.

Yapko, M.D. (1992). *Hypnosis and the Treatment of Depression*. New York: Taylor & Francis.

Yapko, M.D. (1996). *Breaking the Patterns of Depression*. New York: Doubleday.

Yapko, M.D. (2003). *Trancework: An Introduction to the Practice of Hypnosis* (3rd edn). New York: Brunner-Routledge.

Zelig, M. & Biedleman, W. (1981). The investigative use of hypnosis: a word of caution. *International Journal of Clinical and Experimental Hypnosis*, 29, 401–412.

Index

Author's Statement

During the almost forty years of my practice of psychotherapy, Subliminal Therapy has become the focus of my profession and my passion in life. My personal objective is to demonstrate the effectiveness of this unusual technique to the conviction of other clinicians, and the public as well.

I believe I have been blessed by the knowledge of how to actually make real and lasting difference in the lives of others, not just with those patients with whom I have had personal contact, but with a great many others through teaching the use of Subliminal Therapy. Questions have been raised about whether the high success I have achieved in my practice is due to my talents or to Subliminal Therapy, and while I would like to claim it to be my talent, talent does not explain the extraordinary effectiveness of Subliminal Therapy; regardless of the talent of the therapist, talent alone cannot explain the results obtained. In verification of this statement, I am currently researching the use of a computerized version of Subliminal Therapy in which, following introduction and instructions, the patient has contact only with the computer. The results are promising.

I conceived the essential concepts of Subliminal Therapy almost forty years ago and have continued to develop and hone the technique since that time. Even at this point, its protocol continues to evolve; yet, it is now sufficiently well-defined to teach to others. I anticipate it will continue to evolve, with the result of increased efficiency and with broadening fields of application; however, thus far it has been pretty much a "one-man show," a situation that must change. In major part, that change will occur as popular demand is created through promotion directly to the public.

I have invested personal funds in establishing the federally approved Subliminal Therapy Institute, Inc., a non-profit corporation, formed for the purposes of researching the effectiveness, promoting and teaching Subliminal Therapy. It is my intention to find funding to accomplish those goals and this book is a necessary step in that direction.

About the Author

Edwin K. Yager, Ph.D., is a Clinical Professor of Psychiatry in the University of California San Diego (UCSD) School of Medicine, and a Staff Psychologist for the UCSD Medical Group. Dr. Yager also maintains a private practice in San Diego, California

Dr. Yager has studied, practiced and taught the clinical use of hypnosis for forty years. He is certified as a Consultant in Hypnosis by the American Society of Clinical Hypnosis and is a Past-President, Fellow and current Board Member of the San Diego Society of Clinical Hypnosis. He offers training privately, under the auspices of the Subliminal Therapy Institute, Inc., the UCSD School of Medicine, and through the San Diego Psychological Association.

In the course of his private practice, Dr. Yager has employed hypnotic techniques, including Subliminal Therapy, in treating several thousand patients who presented a wide variety of psychological, as well as psychogenic physical problems.